Psychogenic
Non-Epileptic
Seizures
PNES

Introduction

Psychogenic non-epileptic seizures (also called psychogenic non-epileptic episodes) include changes in movement, feeling, or consciousness that resemble epileptic seizures but are not caused by abnormal electrical activity in the brain (PNEE). Nonetheless, PNES represents the exterior manifestation of internal issues like stress, trauma, or emotional problems. PNES may be tricky to identify as its symptoms match those of epileptic seizures but are insensitive to antiepileptic therapy.

Video electroencephalography (EEG) monitoring, which may assist in differentiating between PNES and epileptic seizures, is one diagnostic tool among several used in making a diagnosis.

Psychotherapy, such as cognitive-behavioral therapy (CBT) or other talk therapy, is often used to treat PNES and assist patients in coping with their emotional pain. Medications such as those used to treat depression and anxiety may also be provided.

Indeed, studies have indicated that people with PNES often have a history of trauma. Any traumatic incident or experience, such as physical or sexual abuse, emotional abuse, neglect, or watching or experiencing a horrific occurrence, may be considered traumatic.

Having encountered trauma is common among those who suffer from PNES:

Those with PNES have a substantially greater probability of having suffered trauma, as indicated by a number of studies. One research, for instance, revealed that 85% of those with PNES also had a history of trauma, the most prevalent forms of which were physical or sexual assault. Another research indicated that those with PNES were twice as likely as those without epilepsy to have experienced childhood trauma and to suffer from PTSD as a result.

It is believed that trauma's potential effects on the brain and neurological system account for the association between the two conditions. Alterations in brain function and structure, such as how the brain processes and reacts to stress, have been linked to traumatic experiences. This may make people more susceptible to diseases like PNES.

Remember that not everyone with PNES has a history of trauma, and not everyone who has experienced trauma will acquire PNES. It is crucial to consider the patient's trauma history while developing a treatment strategy for PNES. Both cognitive behavioral therapy (CBT) and eye movement desensitization and reprocessing (EMDR) are effective trauma-specific therapies that have been demonstrated to reduce PTSD symptoms and rates (PNES).

Chapter 1

What is Psychogenic non-epileptic seizures (PNES)

Which demographics are most vulnerable to PNES effects?

Every person, regardless of age, gender, or race, may be diagnosed with PNES. However, research shows that PNES is more often diagnosed in women than males and that those with a history of trauma or other mental health issues are at a greater risk of acquiring PNES.

Moreover, the studies above demonstrate that PNES often co-occurs with other mental health problems such as anxiety, depression, and PTSD (PTSD). Individuals with a neurological disorder or epilepsy history are also at a greater risk for PNES.

It's crucial to remember that people with PNES don't knowingly or willingly create their symptoms. PNES is an actual medical illness that has to be diagnosed and treated with compassion and a team approach.

Potential risk factors for progressive neuroendocrine sclerosis are:

- One's history of physical or emotional neglect or abuse, or even sexual abuse, in the past.
- Mood disorders, PTSD, and personality problems are often seen together.
- The act of suppressing or covering up one's emotion.

Due to greater exposure to trauma, PNES is also more common among veterans than among the general population.

What percentage of people experience PNES?

PNES's prevalence is unclear, according to the available research. Yet, PNES is incorrectly diagnosed as epilepsy in 20% to 40% of patients who see epilepsy experts with intractable (untreatable) episodes.

If you have PNES, what do you do?

In some instances, the outward signs of PNES (psychogenic non-epileptic seizures) might be similar to those of epileptic seizures. Unlike epileptic seizures, which are triggered by abnormal electrical activity in the brain, PNES have no such cause.

Physical symptoms:

The following are some examples of typical physical manifestations of PNES:

- In some people with PNES, convulsions occur, which may look a lot like epileptic seizures.
- Some people with PNES may have a loss of consciousness during their seizures.
- Weakness or paralysis of the muscles; PNES may cause this, and it can affect any or all of your muscles.
- Possible PNES side effects include tremors and shaking.
- Numbness, tingling, and the sensation of pins and needles are among the sensory symptoms that PNES might bring on.
- Breathing problems: Some people with PNES report having trouble breathing during seizures.
- Both epileptic and non-epileptic convulsions have been linked to incontinence and a lack of bladder control. The powerful muscular spasms that follow an epileptic seizure might cause a loss of bladder control. The bladder may constrict and empty spontaneously as a result of this. Incontinence and lack of bladder control may occur in non-epileptic seizures, commonly known as psychogenic non-epileptic seizures (PNES). However, the process is different since PNES are not brought on by irregular brain electrical activity. Anxiety or fear may set off a PNES, and in some situations, this can lead to a loss of

bladder control. There are a variety of medical diseases besides UTIs, bladder issues, and neurological abnormalities that may lead to incontinence and loss of bladder control. A medical expert can only determine an accurate diagnosis and treatment plan; therefore, you must seek one out if you have any of these symptoms.

Psychological symptoms:

Epileptic and non-epileptic seizure sufferers often endure emotional anguish and worry in the hours leading up to and after their seizures.

- Anxiety and mental discomfort may be a precursor to an epileptic seizure, known as an aura. The nervousness may be due to the brain's undergoing changes in preparation for the episode, which might make it more challenging to deal with the upcoming event. Confusion and disorientation are expected during the postictal state (the time following a seizure) and may cause emotional anguish for someone who has just had one. Anxiety and mental discomfort may be a precursor to an epileptic seizure, known as an aura. The nervousness may be due to the brain's undergoing alterations in preparation for the attack. Seizure survivors typically struggle emotionally in the postictal state because of the disorientation and bewilderment commonly following a seizure. Many people who suffer psychogenic non-epileptic seizures report feelings of dissociation or isolation from their environment (PNES). Anxiety, emotional trauma, and dissociation are the psychological roots of PNES, not aberrant electrical activity in the brain.

- A person who is dissociated from their environment may feel as if they are viewing themselves from a distance or as though they and their surroundings don't exist at all. This emotional distance might be a coping tactic for dealing with intense feelings of stress or trauma. Dissociation is a possible side effect of a PNES. During a seizure, the person may experience a loss of consciousness and bodily control. After an episode, a person's mental state might become clouded, and they may feel bewildered or detached from their environment.

- Many people suffer from memory loss or disorientation after having a seizure, epileptic or otherwise. The postictal state, which occurs after an epileptic seizure, is associated with memory loss and disorientation. Confusion, disorientation, and memory loss are all possible during the postictal state, which may last a few minutes to many hours. This may result from both the physical and mental tiredness that usually follows a seizure and the consequences of the outbreak itself. Confusion and memory loss are also possible after having a non-epileptic seizure, sometimes called a psychogenic non-epileptic seizure (PNES). Psychological variables, including worry or emotional stress, are the true culprits behind PNES rather than aberrant electrical activity in the brain. Those who have just recovered from a PNES may feel disoriented and confused and may even forget what happened during the seizure.

- Many people who have suffered trauma or who suffer from anxiety disorders report feeling hypervigilant or always on guard. In addition, certain forms of seizure, such as psychogenic non-epileptic seizures, include this symptom (PNES).
- During a seizure, one may have hypervigilance, a heightened awareness of one's environment and possible dangers. The "fight or flight" reaction, triggered by the sympathetic nervous system, may be to blame. Auras and warning signs may sometimes be experienced before a seizure, and hypervigilance has been linked to being one of them. Anxiety and emotional distress may contribute to hypervigilance in people with PNES. Maybe as a defense strategy against harm, some people have evolved a heightened awareness.

It's worth noting that some people with PNES have no physical symptoms during seizures, while others may suffer a broader range of symptoms. A medical expert is needed to make a correct diagnosis and decide on a course of therapy.

Signs of attacks:

Observation alone cannot tell doctors if a patient is suffering a PNES episode or an epilepsy-related seizure, although the following signs of an attack strongly imply PNES:

- Outbreaks of the explosive kind that last longer than ten minutes.

- Involuntary convulsions accompanied by full consciousness.
- Head jerking quickly from side to side.
- Discordant limb motion.
- Inability to respond; eyes closed.
- Hip thrusting.
- Shifting motion habits.

People with PNES often have additional mental symptoms or diagnoses, such as depression or panic attacks, since PNES is linked to psychiatric illnesses.

Where does PNES come from?

Understanding the cause of PNES is crucial for several reasons:

There are several reasons why it's essential to figure out what triggers PNES (Psychogenic Non-Epileptic Seizures):

The first step in providing patients the treatment they need is establishing that their symptoms are caused by PNES rather than epileptic seizures. Medication used to treat epilepsy is ineffective for PNES; therefore, a wrong diagnosis might lead to unnecessary and hazardous therapy.

Individualized care: Doctors can better assist patients with PNES if they know what's causing the condition. Psychotherapy for underlying mental health issues, stress management techniques and medication for co-occurring illnesses are all potential treatments for epilepsy.

Better patient results may be achieved by delving deeper into the root causes of PNES, allowing for a more thorough and tailored approach to therapy. This can lessen the occurrence and severity of seizures, raise the quality of life, and reduce the need for medical treatment.

PNES seizures may be avoided in certain circumstances by identifying and treating the underlying causes and risk factors. For instance, those particularly vulnerable to PNES may be able to prevent its onset if they get early treatment for stress or trauma.

Accurate diagnosis, individualized treatment, better patient outcomes, and prevention all hinge on a firm grasp of the factors that give rise to PNES. Healthcare providers may provide patients with PNES the best care possible by using a multifaceted approach to diagnosis and therapy that considers the disorder's many different causes.

Factors responsible for PNES:

A lack of social connections and emotional support:

Although heightened stress and emotional discomfort promote seizures, social connection and a lack of emotional support are risk factors for PNES (Psychogenic Non-epileptic Seizures). Isolation from others and a lack of social support might increase one's risk for PNES in the following ways:

- Stress Levels Rising: Loneliness and isolation, which may raise stress levels, might result from a lack of social interaction and support. Individuals with PNES are more susceptible to having seizures triggered by stress due to the physiological changes that stress may cause.
- A lack of coping tools might make it difficult for people with PNES to deal with stressful situations and difficult emotions. People with PNES may find it challenging to cope with the mental and emotional issues that contribute to their seizures if they do not have access to these supports.
- Depression, anxiety, and despair are all bad feelings that may develop when people feel alone and unsupported. People with PNES are more likely to have seizures while experiencing these feelings because they are associated with brain alterations that promote seizure activity.
- Individuals with PNES may have a more difficult time accessing healthcare due to social isolation and a lack of support systems. The illness may worsen due to a lag in diagnosis and treatment.

A lack of social connection and support may raise the likelihood of PNES by heightening the experience of stress and emotional discomfort, diminishing the availability of coping mechanisms, and amplifying the intensity of negative feelings. Medical experts must address these social aspects as part of an all-encompassing strategy for treating PNES. Working with family and carers to offer a supportive atmosphere may include linking those with PNES to support groups or counseling services.

Family dynamics and relationship issues:

Some people have PNES (Psychogenic Nonepileptic Seizures) due to family dynamics or interpersonal problems. To what extent might family and interpersonal issues play a role in the onset or worsening of PNES?

- Individuals with PNES may experience increased stress due to interpersonal conflict, including arguments or tense family situations. Since stress is a recognized trigger for PNES, it may increase the probability of seizures.
- Personal or familial history of trauma or abuse: Some people acquire PNES because of their own or a close relative's experience with trauma or abuse. Seizures are more common after traumatic brain injury, and other mental illnesses may contribute to PNES.

PNES may also emerge through dysfunctional patterns of communication within the family. A seizure may be triggered by several factors, including stress and mental discomfort, neither of which can be alleviated if these things aren't dealt with.

- Isolation and despair are common reactions to the emotional discomfort caused by PNES, and not having the support of loved ones may amplify these sentiments.
- The stress of a child's or adolescent's parents or primary carers may have a role in the onset or worsening of a pediatric neuroendocrine syndrome (PNES). A child's or adolescent's heightened sensitivity to their parents' emotional distress may cause them to have an outburst that causes a seizure.

Stress, a history of trauma or abuse, changes in family communication, and a lack of social support are all ways in which family dynamics and interpersonal problems may lead to the onset or worsening of PNES. Clinicians treating patients with PNES should consider these considerations when designing a treatment plan. This may include family therapy, counseling, or carer support groups.

Cultural factors:

Cultural influences may influence PNES (Psychogenic Nonepileptic Seizures) in several ways. Such instances are as follows:

- A social stigma may be attached to PNES and other mental health disorders in various cultural contexts. The illness may worsen if people are reluctant to seek therapy or put off going to the doctor because they fear being judged negatively.

- Cultural ideas about the origins and management of sickness and seizures may influence individuals' and their families' reactions to PNES symptoms. Certain cultures, for instance, may look upon seizures as evidence of possession or divine retribution, leading them to believe that spiritual or traditional healers are required instead of medical intervention.
- Stress may be affected by cultural norms and expectations about one's profession, family, and social obligations, and these variables may play a role in the onset of PNES in vulnerable people. The risk of developing PNES is higher in women than in males, and this may be due, in part, to societal expectations about women's roles as carers for family members.
- Delays in diagnosing and treating PNES may occur because certain cultures have less access to medical care than others. This may worsen the problem and lead to other health complications.

Individuals' and their families' understanding of PNES symptoms, as well as their access to treatment, may be influenced by cultural variables. Clinicians caring for patients with PNES should be culturally competent. They are aware of and sensitive to patients' backgrounds and values and can incorporate such perspectives and experiences into developing individualized treatment regimens. This may include collaborating with community leaders to lessen the stigma associated with mental health issues or integrating traditional healing techniques into treatment strategies.

Neurobiological Mechanism:

PNES, or psychogenic non-epileptic seizures, have not yet fully elucidated their precise neurobiological causes. However, many ideas and research have pointed to potential neurobiological elements in the development and maintenance of PNES.

- Researchers have shown that people with PNES may be more susceptible to seizures due to abnormal cortical excitability. Changes in neurotransmitters, ion channels, or other physiological processes might lead to this increased excitability.
- Those who suffer from PNES often struggle to control their emotions, which is known as emotional dysregulation. Many studies have pointed to problems in the brain circuits responsible for emotion regulation as a possible cause of PNES. PNES patients have been shown to have anomalies in many brain areas, including the amygdala and prefrontal cortex, both of which play essential roles in emotional regulation.
- Mental health issues Anxiety, sadness, and trauma have all been linked to the onset of PNES. Seizures may be triggered by brain structure and function changes, which the earlier variables may influence.
- Research has shown that people with PNES may have abnormal brain connections, which may play a role in initiating and maintaining seizures. For example,

people with PNES have been shown to have anomalies in the default mode network, a set of brain areas involved in self-referential thought and emotion regulation.

Studies have suggested that alterations in cortical excitability, disruptions in emotion regulation, psychological factors, and altered brain connectivity may contribute to the development and maintenance of PNES. However, the exact neurobiological mechanisms responsible for PNES are not fully understood. A better grasp of these neurobiological aspects may aid in designing more efficient therapies for people with PNES.

Congenital Brain Malformations:

Psychogenic non-epileptic seizures are characterized by their resemblance to epileptic ones but lack a biological basis (PNES). There is mounting evidence linking PNES to alterations in brain anatomy and function.

Grey matter volume in the anterior cingulate cortex and insula, two brain areas important for emotion regulation and interoception, was lower in patients with PNES. In addition, the default mode network, which governs self-referential cognition and mental wandering, has been shown to have increased functional connectivity in people with PNES.

Based on our evidence, trauma or stress may contribute to the development of PNES. Trauma may alter the hypothalamic-pituitary-adrenal (HPA) axis, which controls the body's response to stress.

The present information implies that anomalies in brain structure or function may be possible risk factors for PNES, while an additional study is required to understand this association completely.

Psychogenic non-epileptic seizures have been linked to genetics and inheritance, according to some research (PNES). Studies have suggested that there may be a family component to PNES; however, the precise genetic pathways involved are still not entirely known.

One research, for instance, determined that first-degree relatives of PNES patients had a 10-fold increased risk of developing the disease compared to the general population. Another study discovered that PNES is more common in families where seizures run in the genes.

Some families may have a combination of environmental and genetic variables at play in the onset of PNES. PNES risk may be raised, for instance, if family members have been exposed to trauma or stress.

Even though further study is required to determine the exact genetic and hereditary components that contribute to PNES, current data shows that there may be a genetic component to the illness and that those with a family history of seizure disorders may be at higher risk.

It is crucial to conduct a comprehensive analysis to isolate and isolate all possible causes and factors:

The development of psychogenic non-epileptic seizures may be attributed to several reasons, some of which may only be identified after a comprehensive evaluation (PNES). Various psychiatric, neurological, and physical conditions may trigger PNES.

The patient's medical history, including a record of previous seizures or other medical disorders, and a complete description of the episodes are essential components of a comprehensive evaluation. A neurological assessment may be required to rule out the possibility of a neurological disorder as the underlying cause of the attacks.

A comprehensive evaluation should include medical but also psychological and environmental aspects that may be involved in developing PNES. Anxiety, depression, and other mental health issues may be ruled out or treated during this process, and the effects of prior trauma or other significant life stresses may be calculated.

An in-depth evaluation may aid in designing an efficient treatment strategy for PNES by revealing any underlying causes and contributing variables. Depending on the person's requirements, this may include a mix of medical and psychological therapies such as psychotherapy and stress management strategies.

Generally, PNES may be better diagnosed and treated if a comprehensive examination is performed on the patient.

Some common mental health issues that may arise together with PNES are:

- Terror Stress Disorder (PTSD).
- Diseases of the depressed mind.
- Disorders characterized by dissociation.
- A condition characterized by manifesting symptoms in non-mental systems.
- Disturbances of personality.

It has been shown that many persons who suffer from PNES also have a conversion condition (also known as functional neurological symptom disorder). The mental illness known as conversion disorder often has physical manifestations. It's because your brain "translates" the impacts of a mental health problem into issues with your central nervous system that you're experiencing these symptoms.

When will we think about the kids?

Adolescents and younger children are also susceptible to developing PNES. In this age range, headaches and stomachaches are more typical psychogenic (stress-induced) symptoms. Most of this manual's advice applies to young and old readers. Triggers in young patients are similar to those in adult patients, except that they are typically less severe and are often related to stresses experienced by more youthful patients, like school or dating. Recovery rates are also higher in children and adolescents.

Should I see a psychiatrist or psychologist?

Some view seeking help from a psychiatrist as evidence of mental weakness or craziness. When it comes to PNES, however, this is not the case. Many patients react negatively when told that their seizures have a psychological cause. Remember that PNES are not manufactured intentionally, so having one is not your fault.

Getting treatment from the person who can help you the most makes the most sense. Psychologists, psychiatrists, and clinical social workers, among others, are trained to spot the psychological causes at play. Sometimes the exact cause of a medical condition is unknown, which is normal.

Still, we'll be able to zero in on the most crucial objective, stopping or at least minimizing the seizures.

In this case, a mental health expert will likely take the lead in caring for you, while your neurologist may still check in on you sometimes. Psychotherapy, stress reduction techniques (including relaxation and biofeedback training), and moral support may all be included into your care to help you cope with the seizures. Antidepressants and other drugs are effective in some instances.

Chapter 2

Diagnosis of PNES

How is PNES diagnosed?

While EEGs are crucial in diagnosing epilepsy, they are often expected in individuals with long-standing epilepsy and should not be used in isolation. Video EEG monitoring that records the symptomatic episodes is the gold standard for confirming a diagnosis of PNES.

It might take a few hours or days for an epileptic seizure to occur during video EEG monitoring. Examination of video and EEG data may help diagnose PNES with high certainty. If a proper diagnosis is made, the patient will likely be sent to a psychiatrist for further treatment.

Yet, with the advancement of technology, video-EEG monitoring may now be performed at the convenience of one's own home and in a hospital.

If a neurologist can't access video-EEG monitoring, cell phone footage from an eyewitness might be beneficial.

Explain how we can be so confident that this is the correct diagnosis?

Electroencephalograms (EEGs) that only take 20 minutes to perform are frequently helpful in diagnosing epilepsy.

It is sensitive enough to pick up on abnormal electrical (epileptic) dis- changes in the brain. However, in patients with confirmed epilepsy, the EEG is frequently normal, so it cannot be used alone to rule out epilepsy.

EEG-video monitoring is the gold standard and is currently the only test for diagnosing PNES. A patient is video and EEG-monitored for several hours to days in the hopes that a seizure will occur. Epilepsy experts can almost certainly diagnose after reviewing the video and EEG recordings. On the other hand, this can only be done if the incidents in question occur frequently enough (once a week or more) to warrant recording. Seizures can be induced using various techniques and then monitored.

My other doctor diagnosed me with epilepsy; why?

Eighty percent or more of PNES patients have Been given antiepileptic medication for a long time before the diagnosis of PNES was made. This does not suggest that your previous epilepsy doctors were less competent than the ones treating you now. Remember that the descriptions of observers, who may miss crucial details, are used to diagnose seizures.

Since EEG-video monitoring requires the expertise of an epilepsy-trained neurologist, it is rarely used in medical practice (epileptologist).

When in doubt, doctors will opt to treat epileptic seizures rather than PNES because of the greater risk associated with the former. If epileptic seizures persist despite treatment, either the diagnosis of epilepsy is incorrect, or the treatment needs to be modified. When this happens, a referral to an epilepsy clinic is sought for a definitive diagnosis.

Why isn't anybody concerned about my odd EEG?

Most people with PNES have been misdiagnosed with epilepsy, as was discussed above. Several others have also had anomalous readings on their EEGs reported. This is because general neurologists' exaggerated interpretations of normal EEG and epilepsy tests are often the source of unnecessary treatment. This is why only trained epileptologists should make a PNES diagnosis.

You should get the actual tracings if your previous EEGs have been abnormal so the specialist (epileptologist) can examine them.

Less than ten percent of PNES patients also have epilepsy. If you have both, you and your loved ones must learn to tell the difference between the two kinds.

What about my abnormal EEG?

Most people with PNES have been misdiagnosed with epilepsy. Similarly,

Several people have had "abnormal" EEG results published. This is because general neurologists' "over-reading" of EEG and epilepsy results in abnormalities when experts would find none. This is why only trained epileptologists should make the diagnosis of PNES.

If you've ever had any abnormalities, your doctor (an epileptologist) would want to see the original EEG tracings. Just around 10% of PNES patients also suffer from seizures. If you have both, you and your loved ones must learn to tell the difference between the two sorts.

Should I seek psychiatric help?

Consequently, as was previously said, PNES (and other conversion disorders) is a mental health issue. Some patients refuse to accept the results of the examination. It's important to remember that PNES is a diagnosed condition with high confidence levels. In contrast to other types of symptoms, psychogenic symptoms are only a "diagnostic of elimination." EEG video surveillance by an epileptologist proves the psychological basis of PNES with about 100% reliability.

Others see seeking help from a psychiatrist as evidence of mental weakness or craziness. Yet, PNES is not the same kind of thing. When informed their seizures are psychological, many patients experience emotional distress. It's essential to remember that PNES aren't manufactured on purpose; thus, it's not your "fault" if you have them.

Making an appointment with the specialist who can assist you the most makes the most sense. Psychologists, psychiatrists, and clinical social workers in the field of mental health are most suited to detect the psychological factors at play. Even if the precise reason is unclear, as with many medical problems, we may still focus on what matters: minimizing or eliminating the seizures.

You may visit your neurologist sometimes, but a psychiatrist or psychologist will be responsible for your care. Seizures may be managed with psychotherapy, stress reduction methods (including relaxation and biofeedback training), and social support.

Analyzing Variables for a Correct Diagnosis:

The diagnosis of psychogenic non-epileptic seizures relies heavily on elimination. Any paroxysmal event, such as syncope, arrhythmia, or other spells, can mimic an attack or PNES. Differential diagnoses may include movement disorders and sleep disorders. Even after ruling out all potential confounding factors, differentiating epileptic seizures from PNES may be difficult. Examples of possible alternative diagnoses for PNES are:

- Lack of convulsions
- Syncope
- Vertigo
- Complex Partial Seizures

Status of early Diagnosis:

It is vital to identify psychogenic non-epileptic seizures as soon as they manifest. The process of arriving at an accurate diagnosis might be lengthy. Psychogenic non-epileptic seizures have a long diagnostic lag time, with a study showing an average of 7.2 years from the beginning of symptoms to a final diagnosis. Many patients with epileptic episodes face severe problems because of inappropriate treatment, such as antiepileptic medication side effects and aggressive, possibly hazardous procedures (such as intubation) for pseudo-status epileptics during emergency room visits.

Confirming that your seizures are not epileptic by getting a proper diagnosis is essential. After getting a correct diagnosis, some individuals say the attacks stopped.

To save money, early detection of psychogenic non-epileptic seizures is crucial. One research indicated that costs associated with treating psychogenic non-epileptic seizures decreased by 84% six months after a diagnosis. There was a drop of 80% in outpatient visits and 97% in ER visits, while costs for diagnostic tests and medications also fell by an average of 76% and 69%, respectively.

Primary care physicians play an essential role in the early detection of psychogenic nonepileptic seizures by referring patients with seemingly intractable seizures to epilepsy clinics. 60% of patients with a new diagnosis of epilepsy have their seizures controlled with a moderate dosage of a single antiepileptic medication, whereas 10% of patients with inadequate management of episodes on the first antiepileptic treatment become rid of attacks (usually the first or second drug used). The patient should be sent to an epilepsy clinic for further evaluation as soon as feasible if their attacks are considered intractable.

Life-threatening consequences result from psychogenic, nonepileptic seizures. Those who have these seizures have a far worse health-related quality of life compared to those who have epilepsy, particularly those who have chronic epilepsy. The adverse side effects of antiepileptic treatment are associated with psychopathology, which contributes to a worse quality of life for patients with psychogenic nonepileptic seizures. Support for early identification of psychogenic nonepileptic seizures, followed by treatment of the underlying mental disorder and, in the absence of accompanying epilepsy, removal from antiepileptic pharmacological therapy, is expanding.

Epidemiology:

About 2/100,000 to 1/30,000 people in the general population may have a seizure not caused by epilepsy each year. This sort of seizure probably occurs often, given the frequency with which MS and trigeminal pain occur. Twenty percent to forty percent of inpatients and outpatients with epilepsy have psychogenic nonepileptic seizures (hospitals and specialty epilepsy centers). Psychogenic nonepileptic seizures affect between 75% and 85% of women. Psychogenic nonepileptic seizures, like conversion disorder, often manifest in young people.

Patients with a history of head trauma, learning impairments, or isolated cognitive deficiencies are at a higher risk of experiencing psychogenic nonepileptic seizures. Patients in this group are more likely to show abnormalities on MRIs and EEGs. These clues point to the possibility that a physical brain disorder contributed to the emergence of these events. Epilepsy-prone patients encounter the same things as those without the condition, such as those who have had a stroke, brain injury, infection, or congenital disability of the central nervous system. Often seen in those with epilepsy affecting the temporal lobe, hippocampal sclerosis affects the hippocampus. It may be more challenging to treat psychogenic nonepileptic seizures if they are difficult to diagnose because of MRI or EEG abnormalities.

While the prevalence of psychogenic nonepileptic seizures in patients with epilepsy ranges from 5% to 60%, this estimate is very variable and depends on the study's methodology and diagnostic criteria.

Just 5-10% of individuals with nonepileptic seizures have concurrent epileptic episodes, according to recent research using strict criteria for the diagnosis of epilepsy.

Etiology:

All forms of psychogenic non-epileptic seizures have an adaptive purpose.

This increases the likelihood that patients with these experiences will resort to unhelpful coping mechanisms when under pressure. In psychogenic non-epileptic seizures, the onset of a stroke is interpreted as a representation of internal psychological conflicts. By cutting off the painful connection to the traumatic event or forbidden emotion, pain tolerance may be increased. So, unlike manufactured disease or malingering, psychogenic non-epileptic seizures are not premeditated but rather emerge as a coping technique to bury traumatic experiences from one's psyche.

There is no one cause for psychogenic non-epileptic seizures; they arise from various interrelated factors. Seizures could originate from psychopathological processes, be a reaction to short-term stress in people who don't otherwise show signs of mental illness, or be a learned behavior in people with impaired cognitive functioning. Psychogenic non-epileptic seizures are a rare manifestation of malingering or factitious disorder.

Patients with psychogenic non-epileptic seizures have a high prevalence of co-occurring psychiatric disorders, with a range of 43%-100% (median: 73.5%). Conditions like PTSD, depression, anxiety, and even conversion, somatization, and dissociation may all be traced back to traumatic experiences. The prevalence of borderline personality disorder is staggering. Dissociative and somatization symptoms are common among people who have psychogenic non-epileptic seizures.

The Complex Etiology of PNES:

Patients' emotional discomfort may have a variety of causes, and this is true for people with PNESs as well as those with any other mental disease. The first step in unraveling the mystery of PNESs is to wonder if specific manifestations can be traced back to underlying emotional difficulties. Several studies have suggested that the degree to which a PNES manifests with motor or affective components is a crucial predictor of long-term success or failure. For instance, patients whose PNESs featured prominent motor components had a lower chance of achieving seizure control, according to one study. Patients who did not exhibit any symptoms during their hospital stay (such as rigidity, shaking, ictal incontinence, tongue biting, PNES status events, or critical care unit admissions) were shown in a second research to have comparable outcomes. Third, research indicated that patients were more likely to be emotionally disturbed if their episodes were characterized by a prevalence of affective rather than motor elements. Although the study wasn't meant to answer this question, the report also suggested that patients with prominently affective components might be more likely to have PNES episodes persist. As a result, there is debate in the published research; the clinical manifestations of PNESs may aid in prognosis in some cases but not others.

Many potential triggers for PNESs have been identified like the many "conversion reactions" described there. The likelihood that any discrete conversion symptom has a unique etiology is poorly understood. One can classify the causes into a few significant classes.

To begin, PNES episodes may develop when the patient or a third party experiences difficulty in social interactions. Some patients, for instance, are more likely to create PNESs, manifested physically as a result of emotional problems, if they have inadequate personalities, adjustment reactions, family conflicts, or have been victims of sexual or physical abuse. A patient's PNES may have been encouraged by those around them. Patients with PNESs can have symptoms of anger management or hatred towards others.

Underlying emotional issues or internal tensions may be the root cause of an incident. This category of reasons includes PTSD, anxiety, panic attacks, OCD, conversion/somatization, and dissociative/depersonalization disorders. Patients, especially those who have simple partial seizures that might develop into PNESs, may, for internal reasons, misread or over-interpret events in their surroundings.

Those with a history of psychosis like schizophrenia are more likely to have PNES episodes. Yet, the kind of psychosis is often not specified in the paper.

Those with PNES may also have mental health issues. These disorders include borderline, histrionic, narcissistic, antisocial, passive-aggressive, avoidant, and passive-dependent. Other probable explanations that match this group include malingering, abnormal conditions, and drug addiction.

There can be a history of brain damage or cognitive issues. Patients with PNESs have been shown in specific research to have a higher risk of MRI or electroencephalogram (EEG) abnormalities and frontal lobe dysfunction.

Finally, other aetiologies, such as those for tic disorders and attention deficit hyperactivity disorder, are discussed in the literature, but they don't easily fit into the schema shown above.

Many factors, including personality and social interactions, may contribute to PNES in any specific individual. As an added complication, a psychiatric diagnosis is elusive for many individuals. These individuals' personalities may be variations, even severe ones, on the norm. PNESs are puzzling since the people experiencing them often seem perfectly healthy. To be explored, however, is the possibility that these individuals will have a favorable clinical outcome.

Chapter 3

PNES in children and adolescents

Epileptic seizures of unknown cause in children and adolescents:

Children and teenagers often struggle with PNES or psychogenic non-epileptic seizures. Because of diagnostic uncertainty, they provide challenges for the pediatrician. On clinical grounds, PNES are often indistinguishable from epileptic episodes. A false diagnosis of epileptic seizures for PNES might have serious repercussions. The costs of unsuitable, unneeded therapies as well as trips to the ER or a hospital, may have a significant impact on a family's finances. Iatrogenic problems may occur due to using unneeded drugs or intrusive procedures, such as intubation, to treat protracted episodes (non-epileptic/pseudo status epilepticus). Interpersonal and familial relationships may suffer as a result of these psychosocial consequences. A misdiagnosis is particularly problematic since it often causes patients to wait longer before receiving necessary mental care, which may negatively impact their prognosis.

Adults have been the focus of several descriptions of PNES. Nonetheless, the field of pediatrics has produced very little body of work. New insights into the causes of PNES and the identification of effective therapies have emerged in recent years.

The majority of this research, however, has only been conducted on PNES-affected people.

Even fewer recent investigations have identified variations in the clinical aspects of PNES between younger children and adolescents, especially concerning the semiology of the episodes and the kinds of stressors.

Prevalence of PNES in children and adolescents:

Adolescents, rather than younger children, are often diagnosed with PNES. It is believed that PNES causes between 2% and 33% of all pediatric seizures in children and adolescents. Differences in research populations, diagnostic criteria, and ascertainment methods are probably to blame for the discrepancy in prevalence estimates.

Females have higher rates of PNES than males. There appears to be a 3:1 to 4:1 female-to-male ratio among PNES cases among young people. In children and adolescents, PNES may manifest at any age. However, it is often identified in preteens (between 12 and 14).

It's vital to remember that children and adolescents may have muddled symptoms and a limited capacity to express their experiences, making it harder to diagnose PNES in them. As a result, medical professionals should be alert for PNES in this group and use reliable diagnostic techniques to separate PNES from epileptic fits.

Importance of understanding PNES in this population:

There are several reasons why it's crucial to have an understanding of psychogenic non-epileptic seizures (PNES) in kids and teens:

Accurate diagnosis: Correct identification is crucial since PNES are often mistaken as epileptic seizures in children and adolescents, resulting in improper treatment and the overuse of antiepileptic drugs. An accurate diagnosis of PNES may save young lives by reducing the need for invasive medical procedures.

Psychological effects: PNES are often linked to psychiatric conditions such as stress, trauma, and anxiety. Better patient outcomes may be achieved when healthcare practitioners are aware of the psychological effects of PNES on children and adolescents and take steps to address these difficulties.

Treatment option: Psychological therapies like cognitive behavioral therapy and family counseling are necessary components of the multidisciplinary approach needed for treating PNES, as opposed to the monotherapy generally used for treating epileptic seizures. Healthcare practitioners may better treat PNES in children and adolescents by considering the disorder's psychosocial and physiological elements.

Education and support: Kids and teens with PNES often need continuing education and help to cope with the disease. Better results and enhanced quality of life may be achieved when healthcare practitioners appreciate PNES and use that knowledge to educate and assist patients and their families.

Accurate diagnosis, treating underlying psychological problems, devising appropriate treatment plans, and providing continuing education and support for patients and their families depend on a firm grasp of PNES in children and adolescents.

The prognosis and long-term outcome of psychogenic non-epileptic seizures (PNES):

Psychogenic non-epileptic seizures (PNES) in children and adolescents have a wide range of potential outcomes depending on factors such as the nature of the underlying psychological problems, the severity of the episodes, and the presence of any comorbid conditions, making it difficult to generalize about prognosis and outcome.

Studies have shown that treatment and management of PNES in children and adolescents may lead to good outcomes such as reduced seizure frequency and intensity, increased quality of life, and better mental health. Mental health methods may be incorporated into the treatment plan. These may include cognitive behavioral therapy, family therapy, and medication.

Seizures and other co-occurring mental health issues, like anxiety and depression, are possible in a subset of children and adolescents with PNES. The length of time that seizures went untreated, a history of physical or sexual abuse, and a lack of social support could all negatively affect the prognosis.

To ensure that patients continue to get the care and treatment they need to manage their illness and achieve the best possible results, it is crucial to conduct regular follow-up care and monitoring. It is also essential to educate patients and their families about and support them through the disease.

Many children and adolescents with PNES have a favorable prognosis and better quality of life with the right therapy and care. However, this varies greatly depending on the specifics of the case.

Effects of PNES, both immediately and over time:

Seizure reduction, improved mood and behavior, and enhanced capacity to deal with stress and anxiety are all potential short-term consequences of psychogenic nonepileptic seizures (PNES) in children and adolescents. Cognitive-behavioral therapy, family counseling, and pharmaceutical therapies are all effective ways to do this.

Variables such as the underlying psychological disorders, the intensity and length of the seizures, and the existence of concurrent illnesses may have a role in the long-term results of PNES in children and adolescents. Possible long-term effects of PNES in kids and teens include:

- Enhanced standard of living: Children and adolescents with PNES may have a better quality of life, fewer symptoms, and an improved capacity to engage in everyday activities with the right therapy and care.
- Reduced anxiety, sadness, and stress are all signs of better psychological well-being that may result from tackling the root psychological disorders related to PNES.
- Children and adolescents with PNES are at a higher risk of acquiring comorbid problems such as depression, anxiety, and behavioral disorders; hence it is essential to take steps to prevent the onset of these diseases. If PNES is diagnosed and appropriately managed, reducing or eliminating the risk of these complications may be possible.
- Reducing healthcare utilization: Hospitalizations, ER visits, and the unneeded use of antiepileptic drugs may all be avoided with proper diagnosis and treatment of PNES.

Depending on the specifics of each case, the long-term effects of PNES in kids and teens may vary significantly. To ensure that patients continue to get the care and treatment they need to manage their illness and achieve the best possible results, it is crucial to conduct regular follow-up care and monitoring.

Chapter 4

Medical and Anatomical aspects of PNES

It may be challenging to distinguish psychogenic non-epileptic seizures from epileptic ones. The consciousness that seems to come and go, trembling that doesn't seem to be in sync with the rest of the body, pelvic thrusting, head jerking to one side, and closed eyes all point to PNES. However, PNES may also be represented by brief periods of sudden unresponsiveness. The patient has been diagnosed with a seizure disorder and is being treated with antiepileptic drugs. Still, there is often a lack of information suggesting a history of non-epileptic seizures or spells from friends or family members.

Even during a chaotic shift, a moment of observation is always taken before any treatment is administered in the emergency room. Procedures in therapy should be carried out first being carefully examined. During a convulsive seizure, the eyes of the patient will usually be open. It is not consistent with epileptic seizures for the eyes to be closed, especially if they are tightly closed, and the person is resistant to opening them during the event. Closing one's eyes during a spell is a reliable indicator of PNES (95% or higher), though there are some outliers.

There is no correlation between seizures and wildly gesticulating, head-swaying, or yelling. If the patient has an epileptic seizure characterized by diffuse cerebral involvement (i.e., four extremities motor movements with episodes), they should be unable to speak during the fit. During the tonic phase of a widespread disturbance, the mouth is typically open; a clenched mouth during this period might prompt suspicion of PNES. Although a person experiencing a generalized epileptic convulsion shouldn't be startled or responsive to stimuli during an episode, PNES may be detected with a short, loud noise or similar startle stimulus. PNES patients may not have the typical postictal phase of tiredness or disorientation that follows generalized epileptic seizures.

These results are not universally accurate, of course. Evidence links frontal lobe epilepsy to behaviors including pelvic thrusting, bicycling, and aberrant posture.

Heart rates of patients experiencing convulsive and non-convulsive seizures of epilepsy were found to be 30% higher than those of patients experiencing non-epileptic events. Nine percent of patients with PNES stutter during an event, which was not seen in patients with epileptic seizures in a single study. In observational studies, researchers found that patients with generalized epileptic seizures experienced postictal deep, noisy breathing, but those with PNES did not.

Thanks to the proliferation of phones with video recorders, eyewitnesses to an event can provide a visual account. The value of analyzing these recordings by expert review in identifying non-epileptic seizures has been demonstrated.

Importance of understanding medical and anatomical factors:

An accurate diagnosis and treatment plan for psychogenic non-epileptic seizures (PNES) need knowledge of these seizures' underlying medical and anatomical causes.

PNES is often misinterpreted as epilepsy; correct diagnosis requires a precise distinction between the two. The absence of electrical abnormalities on electroencephalography (EEG) in PNES and the presence of psychosocial stresses are two examples of the medical criteria that help to differentiate PNES from epilepsy and are necessary for this.

Secondly, it is helpful to have a working knowledge of the anatomical causes of PNES to guide therapy. There is speculation that the limbic system, the prefrontal cortex, and the autonomic nervous system all have a role in developing PNES. To better treat each patient, we must understand the underlying neurobiological pathways that cause PNES.

Finally, dispelling myths and misunderstandings about PNES is facilitated by education on the subject's medical and anatomical aspects. Given the high prevalence of co-occurring mental disorders such as despair and anxiety, the stigmatizing label of "faker" or "attention seeker" may devastate people with PNES. Reducing this stigma and improving patient outcomes may be accomplished by educating healthcare providers and the general public about the medical and anatomical foundations of PNES.

For proper diagnosis, appropriate treatment, and the mitigation of social stigma, knowledge of the underlying medical and anatomical elements contributing to PNES is essential.

Overview of brain anatomy relevant to PNES:

Seizures of this kind, called PNES, result from a combination of psychological and biological causes, including the brain's structure. A summary of PNES-related brain anatomy is as follows.

A network of brain regions responsible for learning and remembering as well as controlling emotions is known as the limbic system. The amygdala, hippocampus, thalamus, hypothalamus, and cingulate cortex make up what is known as the limbic system. Research suggests that PNES may be caused, at least in part, by emotional processing and memory changes brought about by dysregulation of the limbic system.

The prefrontal cortex plays a role in executive functions, including decision-making, planning, and regulating impulses. Deficits in cognitive control and emotional regulation are hallmarks of PNES, and studies show that changes in prefrontal brain activity may contribute to this.

The autonomic nervous system controls the heart, blood pressure, and digestive processes. Changes in heart rate variability, breathing, and other physiological processes may indicate that autonomic nervous system dysregulation is involved in the genesis of PNES.

The basal ganglia are a collection of brain regions that regulate movement and acquire new skills via reinforcement learning. Changes in motor control and habit formation, in particular, have been linked to PNES, suggesting a role for dysregulation of the basal ganglia in its development.

The frontal-subcortical circuitry is a set of neural pathways in the brain that control movement, emotion, and thought. PNES has been linked to disruptions in this circuitry via shifts in attentional focus and motor control.

PNES-related brain architecture is complex and includes several brain areas and networks. Further study is required to thoroughly understand the neurobiological underpinnings of PNES and its relationship to psychological and social aspects.

Role of limbic system in PNES:

The limbic system and the prefrontal cortex are essential players in psychogenic non-epileptic seizures (PNES) etiology.

The limbic system is a collection of brain regions responsible for regulating and storing our emotions and learning and remembering. The current body of research suggests that issues in the limbic system may play a role in the development of PNES. Studies show that those with PNES had increased amygdala activity, which is essential since the amygdala is a critical element of the limbic system involved in processing emotional information. This heightened activity may cause heightened emotional reactions, setting off PNES. Seizures are exacerbated by alterations in the limbic system, which may be brought on by trauma and stress linked to the onset of PNES.

The function of the Prefrontal Cortex:

Higher-order cognitive activities including decision making, planning, and impulse control all take place in the prefrontal cortex of the brain. It has been hypothesized that PNES is linked to anomalies in the prefrontal brain. For example, research has indicated that persons with PNES had lower prefrontal brain activity, especially in cognitive control and emotion regulation areas. This diminished activity may lead to difficulty in managing emotional reactions, which might precipitate PNES. Moreover, defects in prefrontal brain function may make it more difficult for persons with PNES to deal with stress and trauma, common triggers for seizures.

Overall, both the limbic system and prefrontal cortex are crucial in emotional and cognitive processing, and anomalies in both areas may lead to the development of PNES. More effective therapies for PNES may be created with knowledge of its underlying neurobiological processes.

Theories on how trauma may contribute to PNES:

There are numerous ideas on how trauma may contribute to the development of psychogenic non-epileptic seizures (PNES) (PNES). Below are some of the most frequently investigated theories:

According to the somatic symptoms hypothesis, people who have been traumatized may use their physical symptoms as a defense mechanism against their overwhelming feelings of emotional misery. Individuals may unwittingly transform their mental discomfort into physical symptoms, which may present as PNES.

According to the dissociation hypothesis, people who experience traumatic events may dissociate from their feelings and body experiences. Those with PNES may exhibit symptoms of dissociation, including a loss of motor control and other bodily signs.

The idea of aberrant brain function proposes that trauma may lead to dysfunction in the brain, especially in regions responsible for emotional processing and regulation. Those with these anomalies may be more prone to developing PNES because they may have trouble controlling their emotional reactions, leading to a greater likelihood of generating physical symptoms.

According to the behavioral reinforcement hypothesis, people who have undergone trauma or abuse may acquire PNES to get attention or avoid negative consequences. Some people with PNES find that they help them deal with their feelings or get them out of sticky situations, so they continue to have seizures even if they know better.

Understanding how trauma increases the risk of PNES is crucial for creating effective therapies for the condition. Individuals with PNES may benefit from treatment targeting trauma resolution, enhanced emotional control, and reduced stress.

Areas for future research in the medical and anatomical aspects of PNES:

Several questions need to be answered regarding the biology and anatomy of psychogenic nonepileptic seizures (PNES). Some of the more exciting directions for future research are as follows:

Neuroimaging methods, including functional magnetic resonance imaging (fMRI) and positron emission tomography, may provide light on the neural mechanisms behind PNES (PET). Future studies might examine alterations in brain activity before, during, and after seizures to zero in on the particular brain regions and networks responsible for PNES formation.

Blood testing and genetic markers are biomarkers that might be used to diagnose PNES and distinguish it from other seizure disorders. Possible directions for further study include the identification of particular biomarkers related to PNES and the creation of novel diagnostic tools that account for biomarker information.

Further randomized controlled trials of therapies for PNES are needed, especially those that aim to address the underlying processes of the condition. The treatment of PTSD in the future may involve a combination of psychotherapeutic methods, such as cognitive behavioral therapy or eye movement desensitization and reprocessing (EMDR), and pharmaceutical procedures, such as those that target specific regions of the brain or particular neurotransmitters.

Research that tracks people with PNES over time may reveal causes for its emergence, its natural course, and the variables that lead to remission or worsening of symptoms. The effects of therapy on the development of the condition over time may also be examined in such research.

Co-occurring mental health conditions, such as anxiety, depression, and post-traumatic stress disorder, are common among those with PNES (PTSD). The link between PNES and these comorbidities may be the subject of future studies, as may the identification of therapies beneficial for PNES and these other illnesses.

The prospect of future study bolsters opportunities for better diagnosis, treatment, and understanding of PNES in the medical and anatomical elements of the condition.

Hope for future therapies based on current studies:

The newest studies on psychogenic non-epileptic seizures (PNES) are shedding light on the disorder's causes and offering new ways to treat it. Several potential novel remedies based on current research are listed below.

- There is growing evidence that virtual reality therapy can help people with PNES. Those receiving VR therapy are put in simulated environments designed to trigger their symptoms so they can learn to control their emotions and behaviors in response to them. Virtual reality therapy has been shown to reduce seizure frequency and improve the overall quality of life in patients with PNES.
- Recent research suggests that mindfulness-based therapies, like MBSR and MBCT, may help reduce

seizure frequency and improve quality of life in people with PNES. This practice is central to learning to recognize and accept one's own internal experiences (thoughts, emotions, and bodily sensations) and being shown how to respond positively to them.

- According to recent research, transcranial magnetic stimulation (TMS), a non-invasive brain stimulation method, may help reduce seizure frequency in people with PNES. Some patients with epilepsy find that transcranial magnetic stimulation (TMS) helps reduce the frequency of their seizures. TMS has shown promise in reducing the frequency of attacks in people with PNES.

- Tools for stimulating or altering neural activity. According to recent research, the frequency of seizures in people with PNES may be reduced by using neuromodulation devices such as vagus nerve stimulation (VNS) and deep brain stimulation (DBS). Stimulating specific regions of the brain or nerves with implanted electrodes has been shown to alter neural activity and reduce the frequency of seizures. Efforts to reduce the number of episodes experienced by people with PNES using vagus nerve stimulation (VNS) and deep brain stimulation (DBS) have met with some success.

New studies on PNES are shedding light on the causes of this condition and pointing the way toward possible new therapies. Some therapies promise to enhance people's lives with PNES, but additional study is required to establish their effectiveness.

Chapter 5

The patient's seizure background

The patient's seizure history is their record of prior fits. Details such as the kind and severity of their seizures, how often they occur, how long they last, any associated symptoms and the results of any diagnostic procedures or treatments they have had are all relevant. To effectively diagnose, treat, manage, and improve a patient's health and quality of life, it is essential to learn about their seizure history. It may aid in the diagnosis of any underlying diseases or risk factors contributing to the seizures and in the formulation of a treatment plan tailored to the patient's specific requirements. Patient interviews, health records, and diagnostic procedures may all be used to piece together a patient's history of seizure disorders.

Importance of understanding a patient's seizure background:

It's crucial to learn about the patient's history of seizures for a few reasons:

The key to efficient treatment of seizures is a correct diagnosis of the underlying disease, which may have a wide range of possible presentations and causes. Medical personnel can better diagnose and treat seizure disorders when they thoroughly understand their patients' seizure histories, including the kind of seizure, any known triggers, and any other contributing variables.

- Methods for Developing a Treatment Plan: Depending on the origin and severity of seizures, many treatment options may be available. Medical personnel can better tailor therapy to the patient's requirements and medical history if they thoroughly understand the patient's seizure history.
- Symptom management: seizures may be distressing for sufferers and their loved ones. Medical personnel may better treat their patient's symptoms and enhance their quality of life by learning about their seizure history.
- Effective seizure management frequently requires a combination of patient education and assistance from medical professionals. By learning about the patient's history of seizures, healthcare providers can better educate and empower the patient in managing their condition.

Knowledge of the patient's seizure history is essential to provide the best treatment possible and improve outcomes for patients with seizures.

Brief overview of different types of seizures:

Many medical issues, not limited to the following, can set off a seizure:

- Recurrent seizures are characteristic of the neurological disorder epilepsy. Many people with epilepsy don't know what causes their attacks, but it could be something as simple as a family history of epilepsy or as complex as a brain injury.
- Several brain injuries, including traumatic brain injury, stroke, and others, can bring on seizures.
- Infections: Meningitis and encephalitis are two infections that can cause seizures.
- Metabolic disorders like hypoglycemia or electrolyte imbalances can bring on seizures.
- Brain tumors can bring on seizures if they grow in the regions of the brain that regulate motor function or sensory perception.

Several aspects of a patient's care depend on discovering the root of their seizures. A few instances of this could be:

- Medication selection: Medications used to treat seizures may differ depending on the cause. Epilepsy-related seizures, for instance, may respond better to certain medications than seizures brought on by brain damage.
- Surgery: If a brain tumor or other structural abnormality in the brain is to blame for the epileptic attacks, then surgery may be an option for treatment.

- Changes in lifestyle, such as a healthier diet and more regular exercise, may be suggested for patients with metabolic disorder-related seizures.
- Epilepsy education: Knowing the root of the problem is critical to controlling symptoms and avoiding further attacks. Patients with epilepsy, for instance, can be guided through identifying potential triggers and learning how to mitigate their effects.

In addition, knowing what triggers seizures is crucial for dealing with any secondary conditions that may crop up. Patients with brain tumors, for instance, may need additional treatment or monitoring to keep cancer under control and prevent further seizures.

To improve patient outcomes and develop a successful treatment strategy, it is essential to identify the underlying cause of seizures.

Several kinds of PNES include:

In contrast to epileptic seizures, which are brought on by abnormal electrical activity in the brain, psychogenic non-epileptic seizures (PNES) originate in the mind. Instead, mental factors like stress and trauma are believed to be linked to PNES. Several distinct forms of PNES exist, each with its presentation and set of distinguishing features:

- Symptoms of a seizure with motor components when a person has a stroke, their muscles may spasm or move involuntarily. These movements' jerky or rhythmic nature may resemble that of epileptic seizures. Although motor seizures in PNES are similar to epileptic ones, they are not accompanied by alterations in brain activity as detected by electroencephalogram (EEG) recording.

- Non-motor seizures can cause various side effects, including altered consciousness, sensory changes, and dissociative symptoms like disconnection from one's body or environment. Pseudo-syncope, or sudden loss of consciousness without the typical motor symptoms of a seizure, can be a symptom of non-motor episodes.
- Mixed seizures: Concurrent motor and non-motor symptoms characterize a mixed seizure. A patient with PNES, for instance, may have a diverse attack characterized by involuntary movements and altered consciousness.

It is crucial to determine the PNES subtype for several reasons:

- Correct diagnosis is essential because PNES are often misdiagnosed as epileptic seizures, which can have severe consequences for treatment and management. Differentiating PNES from epileptic seizures and giving patients the correct treatment depends on knowing the type of PNES they have.
- Planning treatment for PNES may necessitate considering the patient's specific type of seizure and any underlying psychological factors exacerbating their condition. Medical professionals can better serve

their patients by determining the type of PNES they are dealing with.

- Patients can learn more about their condition and how to cope with symptoms if they are educated about the different types of PNES. To lessen the frequency and severity of their seizures, patients with motor seizures, for instance, may find that learning relaxation techniques are helpful. Correctly diagnosing and treating PNES requires first narrowing down the possible causes to a specific type. Patients may have better outcomes and experience less disruption to their daily lives as a result of this.

Importance of obtaining a patient's medical history:

Assessing a patient's health requires gathering relevant information about the person's past medical conditions and treatments. The patient's current and previous medical issues, as well as their family medical history, lifestyle choices, and prescriptions and supplements, are all part of the information that has to be gathered for this step. Some of the main reasons why it is crucial to get a patient's medical history are as follows:

- Correct diagnosis: information from a patient's medical history may help understand the patient's present health and rule out or diagnose potential causes for the patient's symptoms. For instance, an individual may be at higher risk for cardiovascular issues if there is a family history of the condition.

- Preexisting conditions and the drugs a patient takes should be considered when creating an individualized treatment plan for each patient. For instance, an alternate treatment plan may be necessary for a patient with a history of allergies or inadequate responses to certain drugs.

- The Measurement of Achievements The ability to monitor a patient's progress and make necessary adjustments to treatment is greatly enhanced by the ability to track changes in the patient's medical history over time. For instance, if a patient's blood pressure or cholesterol levels suddenly fluctuate, this could mean that they need to make changes to their medication or way of life.

- Healthcare providers can learn about patients' risk factors and potential health problems by reviewing their medical records. For instance, a patient with a strong family history of colon cancer may benefit from routine screenings for the disease.

- Educating patients about their health risks and how to manage their conditions requires a thorough understanding of the patient's medical history. A patient with a history of diabetes, for instance, might gain from education on how to better manage their blood sugar levels through various healthy lifestyle choices.

To provide proper care, collecting relevant information about the patient's health history is necessary. It helps doctors diagnose patients' conditions, create personalized treatment programs, and inform their patients about potential dangers and preventative measures.

Medical conditions that may impact seizure treatment and management:

Seizures can be difficult to treat and manage because of the various underlying medical issues affecting their administration. The following are examples of some of the most prevalent medical problems:

- Seizures and their treatment and management can be affected by neurological conditions like multiple sclerosis, Parkinson's disease, and stroke.
- Seizures and the chance of developing epilepsy can result from traumatic brain injury (TBI). TBI-related seizures may respond to treatment with antiepileptic drugs or other methods.
- Tumors of the brain can trigger fits by interfering with the brain's typical electrical activity, leading to convulsions. Seizures caused by a brain tumor may be treated with surgery, radiation therapy, or medication.
- Seizures can be brought on by brain inflammation, which is triggered by infections like meningitis and encephalitis. Antibiotics or antiviral medication may be prescribed to treat the underlying condition, and antiepileptic drugs may be used to control seizures.
- Metabolic disorders: Electrolyte or blood sugar imbalances and hypoglycemia are among the metabolic conditions that can bring on seizures.

Medication for epilepsy and therapy for the underlying metabolic disorder may be necessary for treatment.

- Seizures and the management and treatment of seizures are affected by psychiatric disorders like depression, anxiety, and post-traumatic stress disorder (PTSD). It is possible that antiepileptic medication, in addition to treating the underlying psychiatric condition, will be neccessary for successful treatment.

Medical professionals assessing a seizure patient should consider these and other related conditions. To improve patient outcomes, gaining insight into the underlying medical conditions contributing to seizures is essential.

Importance of Patient's education and self-management:

While dealing with seizures, patient education and self-management are crucial. Improved quality of life, decreased frequency and intensity of attacks, and prevention of consequences may all result from people being better informed about their disease and how to manage it.

Here are a few examples of why patients must learn how to manage their health:

Improved comprehension: Patients taught about their illness have a better grasp of its causes, triggers, and treatment options. This may help them feel more in command of the situation and lessen the stress and worry of having seizures. Increased compliance with prescribed medication regimens is associated with fewer adverse drug reactions and fewer seizures in patients with a firm grasp of their treatment plans.

Seizure management through lifestyle changes: Patients can learn how to change their lifestyle, such as getting enough sleep, avoiding triggers, and following a healthy diet, to aid in seizure management. By making some of these changes, you can lessen the severity and frequency of your seizures and boost your general health.

Emergency preparedness: Emergency preparation involves informing patients of their options in the case of an emergency, such as how to handle seizures at home and when to seek professional help.

Improved communication with healthcare providers: Patient education leads to better communication with doctors and better treatment results.

Patients who have epilepsy must be taught how to take charge of their condition and manage their symptoms on their own. A patient's quality of life may be significantly enhanced by their healthcare professionals' efforts to educate them about their illness and encourage self-management, which has been shown to decrease seizure frequency and severity.

Chapter 6

What is the difference between Epilepsy and PNES?

Importance of differentiating between epilepsy and psychogenic non-epileptic seizures (PNES):

There are several reasons why it's crucial to differentiate between epilepsy and psychogenic non-epileptic seizures (PNES):

- Patients must obtain an accurate diagnosis to begin therapy as soon as possible. A wrong diagnosis might cause you to take medicine you don't need, cause unpleasant side effects, and delay getting the required therapy.
- Variable Medical Interventions: The therapies for epilepsy and PNES are different. Antiepileptic medications (AEDs) and, in rare situations, surgery are used to treat epilepsy. Psychological therapies, including CBT, hypnotherapy, and psychotherapy, are the mainstays of treatment for PNES.

- Many factors contribute to the prognosis of epilepsy and PNES; hence a proper diagnosis is essential for making an informed prognosis. As compared to epilepsy, PNES has a better prognosis since patients are more likely to improve or go into remission when given the proper medication.
- Emotional and social effects Individuals with epilepsy and PNES may experience unique difficulties in these areas. Individuals with epilepsy may encounter prejudice and stigma if their disease is seen as a neurological issue. In contrast, those with PNES may experience denial or misunderstanding from loved ones if their condition is seen as psychological.

Knowing the difference between epilepsy and PNES may help with diagnosis, treatment, prognosis, and coping with either illness's social and emotional effects.

Comparison between Epilepsy and PNES

There are some parallels between epilepsy and PNES (Psychogenic Non-Epileptic Seizures), despite these two illnesses having different origins and treatments. Examples of this are:

- Physiological manifestations of PNES and epileptic seizures may have similar outward appearances. Similar symptoms, such as fainting, loss of consciousness, and convulsions or jerking motions, have been linked to both disorders.

- The emotional and psychological variables that might bring on these diseases are comparable.
- Quality of life in many areas, including social, emotional, and professional spheres, may be negatively affected by epilepsy and PNES.
- Both epilepsy and PNES need correct diagnosis and treatment to control symptoms and enhance the quality of life.

These ailments have specific symptoms, but they are still quite different diseases with very other root causes and treatments, and they need the attention of doctors who specialize in each of those areas.

Epilepsy VS PNES:

Despite the similarities in presentation, epilepsy and psychogenic non-epileptic seizures (PNES) are classified and treated differently. Some important distinctions between epilepsy and PNES include the following:

Different from epilepsy, which is a neurological ailment triggered by irregular brain electrical activity, PNES is a psychological syndrome characterized by seizures unrelated to electrical activity in the brain.

Stress, lack of sleep, bright lights, and even certain drugs may all bring on a seizure in someone with epilepsy. The opposite is true with PNES seizures, often brought on by mental or emotional strain.

An electroencephalogram (EEG) may reveal irregular brain electrical activity during and between episodes in people with epilepsy. The EEG is frequently normal in PNES.

Several seizures may occur in epilepsy, including tonic-clonic, absence, and complex partial seizures. In contrast, PNES seizures are not always easily identifiable as one form of epileptic seizure but might manifest in various ways.

In many cases, anti-convulsant drugs may be used to manage the seizures associated with epilepsy, however, this is not the case for those with post-neuronal excitability syndrome (PNES). Instead, psychotherapy is often used to treat PNES to address the psychiatric origins of the seizures.

Epilepsy is a lifelong disorder that needs constant attention from medical professionals, but PNES responds well to treatment and often has a brighter outlook.

PNES is not a deliberate action but an unconscious reaction to emotional or mental strain. Treatment for epilepsy and PNES are pretty different; thus, a correct diagnosis is crucial.

Because of this, it is crucial to see a doctor to get a proper diagnosis and treatment.

Common misconceptions about PNES:

Misconceptions and misunderstandings often surround psychogenic non-epileptic seizures (PNES), a seizure condition. Misconceptions concerning PNES often include the following:

Unlike epileptic seizures caused by aberrant brain activity, PNES seizures are not usually believed to be "genuine" seizures. Yet, PNES-induced convulsions are genuine and might be devastating for the patient. With the advancement of technology, video-EEG monitoring may now be performed at the convenience of one's home and in a hospital.

Another common myth that might lead to discrimination against persons with PNES is that it is a type of malingering or faking. PNES is characterized by involuntary convulsions brought on by emotional or mental stress.

PNES indicates mental disorder or frailty: Seizures caused by PNES are a symptom of emotional distress rather than a sign of mental illness. Many people with PNES also have a history of trauma or another mental health disorder.

PNES is simple to regulate: This misconception can be very frustrating for those who suffer from PNES. PNES cannot be managed with anti-convulsant drugs in the same way that epilepsy is. Psychotherapy is frequently used to treat PNES to address the psychiatric factors contributing to seizures.

Contrary to popular belief, PNES are not uncommon. Researchers have found that as many as 20% of patients referred to epilepsy centers for evaluation of seizures have PNES.

To properly diagnose and treat PNES, it is crucial to recognize that it is an accurate and intricate disorder. It is important to dispel these myths to improve the lives of people with PNES and lessen the stigma associated with the condition.

Preventing and correcting common misunderstandings concerning PNES:

Many methods exist for combating misinformation and lowering prejudice towards those who live with PNES:

- One of the best methods to combat misinformation and stigma is raising public understanding through educational campaigns. Accurate information regarding PNES may be provided by healthcare providers, advocacy groups, and community organizations.

- Honest and honest communication may help eliminate confusion and increase familiarity with PNES. It can lessen prejudice and increase compassion by encouraging people with PNES to speak out about their experiences.
- The terminology used to explain PNES may also help lessen people's negative connotations about the condition. Promoting understanding and decreasing unfavorable attitudes towards persons with PNES may be aided by using neutral and non-judgmental language.
- Groups that bring together those who understand what it's like to live with PNES may greatly help those dealing with the condition alone or with loved ones. People may open up, get support, and gain insight from one another in these groups.
- Advocacy: Advocacy may aid in disseminating information about PNES and advancing the rights of those who suffer from it. Advocacy work may take the form of many different things, such as pushing legislation that helps people with PNES, campaigning for research funding, or spreading awareness via public events and campaigns.
- Individuals with PNES may benefit from less stigma and increased community understanding if they are included in community activities. People with PNES may benefit from being encouraged to join in on local events and activities that unite the community.

Education, communication, language, support, advocacy, and inclusion are just some ways to overcome stigma and misunderstandings about persons with PNES. Together, we can improve the world for people with PNES by spreading awareness and eliminating discrimination.

Chapter 7

How does PNES affect me?

What effects does PNES have on me?

Everyone, regardless of age, gender, or race, is at risk for developing PNES. Studies reveal that PNES is more likely to be diagnosed in women than males and that those with a history of trauma or other mental health issues are at a greater risk of acquiring PNES.

And as the studies mentioned above demonstrate, PNES is often associated with other mental health concerns, including anxiety, melancholy, and post-traumatic stress disorder (PTSD). A history of epilepsy or other neurological disorders may also increase the likelihood of developing PNES.

It's crucial to remember that the person experiencing PNES is not responsible for creating them on purpose. PNES is an actual medical illness that has to be diagnosed and treated with compassion and a team approach.

Impacts of PNES on daily life:

Psychogenic non-epileptic seizures, or PNES, can have severe consequences for one's daily life. Some of how PNES might influence a patient are as follows:

- Effects on the body: PNES can bring on physical symptoms like epileptic seizures, including a loss of consciousness, muscle spasms, and trembling. These physical manifestations can be distressing and tiring and can also lead to harm if the affected person falls while having a seizure.
- Those affected emotionally by PNES and their loved ones may find the symptoms upsetting and challenging to understand.
- When others view the seizures as "fake" or "attention-seeking," the person with PNES may experience stigma, guilt, and social exclusion.
- The ability to hold down a job, attend classes, or engage in extracurricular activities may all be impacted by PNES, all of which have social repercussions. When people fear having a seizure in front of others, they may avoid going out in public or even stop going to work.
- Expenses associated with hospitalizations, diagnostic tests, and medications can all rise due to PNES. Another source of financial loss is time lost from work or school as the individual deals with their condition.
- Having PNES can put a strain on your relationships with loved ones. Loved ones can grow frustrated or resentful if they cannot comprehend the severity of the patient's condition.

- An individual experiencing a seizure while behind the wheel poses a threat to himself and other motorists. It is recommended that many patients with PNES wait until their episodes are under control before getting behind the wheel.
- The physical health of a person with PNES may be negatively impacted in several ways. A person's capacity for physical activity and general physical health may suffer.

PNES can severely disrupt daily life. Still, with treatment and support, many people find they can manage their symptoms and even experience an improvement in their quality of life.

Risks associated with PNES:

To clarify, PNES are a kind of seizure not triggered by aberrant electrical activity in the brain but rather by psychological variables like stress, worry, or trauma. PNES, albeit upsetting and disruptive, are usually not life-threatening.

Nonetheless, PNES is not without its hazards, which might have severe consequences for the patient. Among them are:

- Unfortunately, PNES is often misinterpreted as epilepsy because of its symptoms. Consequently, proper therapy for underlying mental health disorders may be delayed while antiepileptic drugs are misused.

- PNES may harm a person's capacity to work and interact socially. This might put a person at risk of feeling alone, down, and anxious.
- Injuries to the body may occur if a person trips and falls during a PNES episode. Bruises, wounds, and broken bones are all possible outcomes.
- Psychological suffering PNES may cause psychological suffering for the one experiencing them and their loved ones. Feelings of humiliation, remorse, and shame may result.
- Potential for injury to oneself: PNES has been linked to cutting and suicidal ideation in certain patients. Anybody having PNES should seek help and get therapy.

Even though PNES are not usually fatal, they may significantly affect a person's standard of living. Anybody struggling with PNES should get the medical and mental health attention they need to control their symptoms and enhance their quality of life.

Mortality in patients with PNES:

In most cases, the risk of dying from having psychogenic non-epileptic seizures (PNES) is low. Patients with PNES have a death rate dissimilar to that of the general population.

While PNES is not a life-threatening illness, it is crucial to highlight that it is linked to several physical and mental health issues that may negatively impact survival rates. Depression, anxiety, and other mental health issues have been linked to PNES and may have severe consequences for patients' physical health.

Increased suicidal ideation and behavior may also be linked to PNES.

In addition, PNES is often mistaken for epilepsy, leading to the inappropriate use of antiepileptic drugs. These drugs can potentially affect a patient's health and well-being due to their potential for adverse effects and drug interactions.

People with PNES must have a proper diagnosis and treatment, including medical and psychosocial assistance. Doing so allows their symptoms to be controlled and further consequences avoided.

Chapter 8

How can I live a normal life?

Strategies for managing PNES symptoms:

When dealing with PNES, several methods might be helpful (Psychogenic Non-Epileptic Seizures). Here are a few examples:

CBT (Cognitive Behavioral Therapy):

Psychogenic non-epileptic seizures differ from epileptic seizures because abnormal brain electrical activity (PNES) does not trigger them. Cognitive behavioral therapy (CBT) may be the most effective treatment for some patients with PNES.

Cognitive behavioral therapy (CBT) emphasizes how one's ideas, feelings, and actions are interconnected. Individuals with PNES may benefit from CBT since it can help them pinpoint the causes of their seizures and work to alleviate those causes.

Cognitive restructuring and behavioral interventions are standard components of CBT for PNES. During the cognitive restructuring, you'll look for and question any limiting assumptions, false beliefs, or other thinking patterns that might trigger your seizures. An individual with PNES may, for instance, feel helpless in the face of their seizures and believe they have no control over them. Through cognitive behavioral therapy, patients may learn to reframe their negative thinking and establish more optimistic and realistic ideas about their abilities to control their seizures.

Exposure treatment, stress management methods, and relaxation exercises are all examples of behavioral approaches used in cognitive behavioral therapy for PNES. Those who cannot control their PNES symptoms may benefit from learning how to practice relaxation techniques. Stress management techniques may teach people how to deal with daily pressures. Those prone to epileptic seizures might benefit from exposure treatment, which entails progressive exposure to conditions known or suspected to bring on episodes.

Individuals with PNES may benefit from CBT by learning more about the psychological aspects contributing to their seizures and acquiring the skills and techniques necessary to control them. It's vital to remember that a licensed therapist with expertise in helping people manage the emotional and psychological effects of seizures should lead any CBT for PNES.

Meditation:

Seizures that aren't epileptic are called PNES, or psychogenic non-epileptic seizures, and things like stress, trauma, or other mental health issues may bring them on. Regular meditation practice may mitigate many of the adverse effects of PNES.

Meditation is an excellent strategy for lowering stress levels, which is a primary contributor to PNES. The stress and tension that might increase the risk of PNES can be alleviated by meditation's calming effects on the mind and body.

Emotional discomfort may cause PNES; however, meditation has been shown to reduce this distress and increase one's capacity to control one's emotions. Those who regularly meditate have a lower risk of developing PNES because they can better identify and manage their feelings when they arise.

Personal insight: PNES patients may benefit from the increased self-awareness of regular meditation. People with PNES may be able to detect triggers better and take action to avoid seizures by raising their awareness of their thoughts, emotions, and body sensations.

Lastly, meditation may have a beneficial effect on PNES by enhancing one's sense of well-being. One way to lessen the impact of PNES is through regular meditation, which has been shown to positively affect one's state of mind and self-perception.

While meditation has shown promise as a treatment for PNES, it is crucial to remember that it is most effective when used with other methods, such as psychotherapy and medication, as prescribed by a medical practitioner.

Sleep:

Sleep is essential for minimizing PNES symptoms and maintaining a regular daily routine. Disturbed sleep habits are associated with PNES, highlighting the significance of sleep to one's health and well-being. People with PNES may benefit from a good night's sleep since it may help them better control their emotions and deal with stress.

These suggestions may help you get a better night's rest:

Follow a consistent bedtime and waketime routine to assist your body's internal clock in adjusting to your needs.

- Develop a soothing nighttime ritual to remind your body it's time to sleep. Some examples of such activities include having a hot bath, reading a book, and engaging in yoga and meditation.

- Make sure your bedroom is dark, cold, and quiet, and use earplugs or a white noise machine to drown out any outside sounds that could keep you awake.
- You won't be able to go to sleep as quickly if you watch TV, use electronics, or have stimulating discussions just before bed.

Because of the potential for coffee and alcohol to disrupt sleep, it is recommended that they be avoided or consumed in much smaller quantities, particularly in the hours preceding bedtime.

See a doctor if you can't go to sleep or stay asleep. They can help you figure out why you're having trouble sleeping and devise a strategy to fix it so you can control your PNES symptoms throughout the day.

Build support system:

Having a solid support system at home is essential for managing PNES symptoms since this disease may be challenging to handle independently. Family, friends, medical experts, and peer support groups are all excellent resources.

Several methods in which assistance may benefit people with PNES are listed below.

- Emotional support: Having someone to speak to and share your thoughts with might be helpful while dealing with PNES, which can be emotionally taxing. Family, friends, and professional counselors are all resources for emotional upliftment. As a result of their illness, people with PNES may need assistance with day-to-day responsibilities, including driving, caring for children, and doing domestic chores.
- Those with PNES may benefit greatly from education and knowledge regarding the disorder and its treatment. Education and information regarding PNES may be obtained from healthcare experts and support groups.
- Support from peers: speaking with those who understand what it's like to live with PNES may help reduce feelings of isolation. Peer support, whether in person or online, may be invaluable.
- To advocate for oneself or another person with PNES is to speak out for their rights and interests to secure adequate services and resources.
- Individuals with PNES should care for themselves by finding social support, practicing stress management, getting enough sleep, and following their healthcare provider's treatment plan. Individuals with PNES may learn to live with their illness and find success with the correct assistance and management approaches.

Physical Exercises:

Physical activity may help manage PNES symptoms since it helps alleviate the tension and worry that can exacerbate the condition. Exercising may help you sleep better, lift your mood, and feel healthier.

For those who suffer from PNES, the following kinds of physical activity have shown promise:

- Walking, running, cycling, and swimming are all examples of aerobic exercises that have been shown to benefit cardiovascular health and mental state. Try to get at least 30 minutes of aerobic activity on most days of the week, preferably more.
- Physical postures, breathing exercises, and meditation are all part of the mind-body practice known as yoga. Reducing tension and anxiety, relaxing muscles, and boosting strength are all possible benefits.
- Tai chi is a non-aggressive martial arts style characterized by relaxed posture, fluid motion, and deep breathing. It has been shown to enhance equilibrium, mobility, and concentration.
- Building strength and muscle tone may be accomplished via resistance training, including weightlifting and bodyweight exercises. Try to get at least two or three bouts of resistance training every week, splitting your time evenly across your main muscle groups.

Individuals with preexisting medical conditions or injuries should see their doctor before beginning an exercise regimen. They may work with you to create a program tailored to your goals and requirements.

To minimize the effects of triggers:

It may be possible to prevent PNES seizures by learning to recognize and avoid their causes. By keeping track of when and where your seizures occur, you may understand better what sets them off, whether it be anxiety, exhaustion, or something else.

Life-Improving Advice:

A better quality of life is possible for those who suffer from psychogenic non-epileptic seizures (PNES), even though this illness might be challenging to manage. Some ideas are as follows:

- Contact a healthcare provider; PNES is a complicated ailment requiring specialized treatment. Obtaining the advice of a trained medical professional specializing in PNES may help you in your quest for knowledge about your problem, identifying potential causes, and creating a workable treatment strategy.
- Learn to deal with stress and emotions more effectively; PNES has been connected to both. Pressure may be reduced, and PNES episodes avoided by regular stress-management strategies, including deep breathing, meditation, yoga, or progressive muscle relaxation.
- You may learn more about your seizures, how often and severely they occur, and how much improvement you've made by keeping a seizure journal. It's

important to discuss any concerns you have with your doctor, and this information might help do so.

- Exercising regularly has been linked to better mental health, lower stress levels, and more happiness. Symptoms of PNES may be alleviated to some degree with low-impact activity like walking, swimming, or cycling.
- Consider joining a support group for persons with PNES to get emotional help, learn from other's experiences, and make connections with others in similar situations.
- To better manage the symptoms of PNES, it is essential to learn effective coping mechanisms, such as positive self-talk, relaxation methods, and visualization.

Remember that learning to control PNES is an ongoing process, and it may take some trial and error to discover the best method(s) for you. Feel free to seek assistance or experiment with other methods.

Chapter 9

Management and Treatment

Overview of medical Treatments for PNES:

Non-epileptic psycho-seizures resemble epileptic convulsions but are not caused by abnormal brain electrical activity (PNES). Instead, it is believed that mental health issues, including stress, worry, and trauma, are to blame.

Often, a multidisciplinary approach is used to treat PNES, emphasizing treating the underlying psychosocial issues that lead to seizures. Several possible medical interventions are listed below.

Pranayama for the PNES:

Mindfulness-based interventions like meditation have positively affected those with psychogenic nonepileptic seizures (PNES). The tension, anxiety, and emotional triggers contributing to PNES episodes may be lessened via reflection, which entails training the mind to concentrate on the present moment.

Individuals with PNES may benefit from a variety of meditation practices, including:

- Mindfulness meditation aims to concentrate on the here and now while also increasing one's awareness of one's own mental and emotional states. This may help people with PNES become more in touch with their bodies and see the precursors of a seizure, perhaps preventing a more severe outcome.
- Meditation on loving-kindness entails sending good thoughts and feelings to oneself and others. Seizure-inducing stress and emotional stressors may be mitigated if this helps people with PNES develop sentiments of compassion and self-acceptance.
- Yoga: The physical postures, breathing exercises, and meditation that make up yoga are beneficial for those with PNES. Empirical evidence shows that yoga may help with stress, anxiety, mood, and sleep.
- Individuals with PNES should work carefully with their healthcare professionals to decide whether meditation is a good therapy choice for them, despite it being typically safe and well-tolerated.
- Individuals with PNES should adhere to their prescription medication and any additional therapies, such as psychotherapy or counseling, that are part of their individualized care plan.

Surgical treatment for PNES:

In most cases, surgical therapies like brain surgery, or deep brain stimulation (DBS) are ineffective in treating PNES since they are not the result of aberrant brain activity.

Surgical treatment is often not suggested for PNES since it does not address the underlying psychological or emotional problems contributing to the seizures.

Yet, in some instances, a structural abnormality in the brain, such as a tumor or a malformation, is to blame for the seizures experienced by PNES sufferers. Surgery to remove the monster may be necessary to minimize the severity and frequency of attacks.

Although surgery may be the only option for PNES treatment in certain circumstances, it is crucial to remember that psychotherapy and counseling are still highly advised as part of a holistic approach. This is because mental variables are typically critical in the emergence and maintenance of PNES, even when a structural abnormality is present.

Because of the lack of attention paid to the potential mental or emotional causes of the seizures, surgical therapy is often ineffective and not indicated for those with PNES. Nevertheless, surgical treatment may be required to ease the attacks in very unusual circumstances if the brain has an underlying anatomical issue. While treating PNES, psychosocial treatments are vital regardless of whether or not surgical intervention is required.

Challenges in management of PNES:

Some variables might make PNES management difficult. Some of the difficulties people may have while trying to control PNES include the following:

- Misdiagnosis: PNES is often misinterpreted as epilepsy due to the similarity between the two conditions' symptoms. This may cause a delay in diagnosis and subpar care.
- In contrast to epilepsy, which is often seen as a neurological condition, PNES is typically seen as a psychological disorder, which may result in social isolation and stigma. Individuals with PNES may shun social interactions and professional chances because they fear ridicule or rejection because of their illness.
- There is currently no gold standard therapy for PNES; therefore, choosing the proper treatment plan may be a frustrating process of trial and error. It's possible that anti-epileptic drugs (AEDs) designed for epilepsy won't help those with PNES.
- Stress, trauma, and other emotional or mental health issues commonly contribute to PNES. Tackling these causes may be difficult and may need ongoing treatment.
- Adjustments to one's way of living may be necessary if PNES is present. The unexpected and distressing nature of seizures means that persons with PNES may need to modify their daily routines, such as avoiding triggers, rearranging their work or school schedules, or cutting down on their activity levels.

- Emotional impact: People with PNES may develop anxiety, depression, and other mental health issues due to the difficulties inherent in living with PNES.

Physical, mental, and social aspects must be considered while treating PNES. It is crucial to have a healthcare team on your side that gets PNES and can tailor their treatment to your specific needs.

How to overcome the challenges of management of PNES:

Similar to epileptic seizures but not produced by aberrant electrical discharges in the brain, PNES (Psychogenic Non-Epileptic Seizures) are a kind of seizure. Instead, it is believed that mental elements, including stress, trauma, and anxiety, have a role in triggering these conditions. Both patients and doctors may struggle with PNES management. Several methods to deal with PNES's management issues are listed below.

- Education: Education's importance for patients and medical professionals cannot be overstated. Patients must be educated on the nature of PNES and how they vary from epileptic seizures. Medical professionals must know PNES and its distinguishing features from epileptic seizures.
- Psychological problems, such as anxiety, sadness, or post-traumatic stress disorder, are common in people

with PNES and may be addressed by counseling (PTSD). Patients may learn to cope with these concerns and decrease the incidence of PNES with counseling and psychotherapy.

- Effective treatment for PNES includes cognitive behavioral therapy (CBT), a kind of psychotherapy. Patients may learn to recognize the negative thoughts, feelings, and actions that precede their seizures and make adjustments to them.
- Medication Although antidepressants and anxiety pills won't help with PNES, they may help people cope with other mental health issues.
- The treatment of PNES calls for a multidisciplinary group effort between a neurologist, a psychiatrist, a psychologist, and a social worker. The patient may be treated thoroughly with the help of specialists from different fields.
- Patients with PNES may benefit from attending a support group because of the emotional support, information, and techniques they can learn there. One way for patients to feel less alone is to join a support group where they may talk to others going through the same thing.
- Care professionals, patients, and their loved ones all need to be able to talk to one another about medical issues. It is essential for patients to feel heard and understood and for healthcare practitioners to be forthright about all aspects of a patient's care, including outcomes and potential side effects.

Yet, with the help of a multifaceted strategy that considers both the physiological and psychological elements of PNES, patients may learn to control their symptoms and enhance their quality of life.

Chapter 10

Recommended types of therapies

PNES Therapy origins and problems:

There are many reasons why it's crucial to gain an understanding of where PNES therapy came from and where it went wrong:

- Improvements in diagnosis are needed because PNES was previously misdiagnosed as epilepsy, which led to inappropriate treatment and poor patient outcomes. Professionals in the medical field can better identify PNES patients and make an accurate diagnosis if they have a firm grasp of the therapy's historical roots.
- Traditional psychoanalytic therapy for PNES has limited empirical evidence for its effectiveness. Patients may have difficulty identifying and addressing underlying psychological factors contributing to their seizures, complicating the development of effective treatments. By recognizing the drawbacks of conventional PNES therapy, medical experts can improve care by incorporating

cognitive-behavioral and mindfulness-based approaches.

- Due to historical misdiagnosis and misunderstanding, patients with PNES may face stigma and skepticism, which must be reduced. Healthcare providers can lessen patient resistance and boost patient outcomes by learning about PNES therapy's roots in the past.
- New methods for diagnosing and treating the disorder can be developed by learning more about the background of PNES therapy and the challenges it has faced over time. Recent progress in the field, for instance, has been made through the application of neuroimaging methods to comprehend better the neural mechanisms underpinning PNES.

Improving diagnosis, developing effective treatments, reducing stigma, and advancing research are all made easier with a firm grounding in PNES therapy's historical roots and issues.

Many factors contributed to the early misdiagnosis and mistreatment of PNES as epilepsy:

Similarity of symptoms: PNES may appear with symptoms comparable to epilepsy, including loss of consciousness, convulsions, and uncontrollable movements. Because of this overlap, diagnosing the two conditions separately was challenging.

Lack of understanding: The psychological elements that might lead to PNES were not well understood in the past. So, it was often believed that a neurological condition like epilepsy was to blame for the fits.

Difficulties in diagnosis: Patients with PNES may not have a clear physical explanation for their seizures, and routine medical testing like an electroencephalogram (EEG) may not reveal any abnormalities.

Misdiagnosis of PNES was also influenced by social and cultural factors, such as the stigma and ignorance surrounding mental health issues. Individuals with PNES were commonly misunderstood and incorrectly diagnosed as malingerers or seeking attention.

Since epileptic drugs and therapies are ineffective for PNES and potentially dangerous, the misdiagnosis of PNES as epilepsy was a significant concern. For people with PNES, a misdiagnosis might mean months or even years without the care they need, resulting in severe impairment and a diminished quality of life.

Healthcare providers can better detect and treat PNES because of improved diagnostic tools and more profound knowledge of the psychological processes leading to the condition.

Early misconceptions and misdiagnosis of PNES as epilepsy:

Although the term "psychogenic non-epileptic seizure" (PNES) was coined in the late 19th century, it wasn't until the 20th century that psychoanalytic theory became the standard method for treating PNES. Early on, doctors commonly misdiagnosed PNES patients as having epilepsy and used ineffective antiepileptic drugs to treat their symptoms.

Sigmund Freud and his followers started investigating the idea that psychological rather than neurological factors may be responsible for certain seizures in the 1920s. According to Freud, PNES is a kind of conversion disease in which the body's response to psychological stress manifests as somatic symptoms. He hypothesized that individuals with PNES were experiencing seizures because they were unable to manage suppressed emotions and that psychoanalysis may help them do so.

In the decades that followed, psychoanalytic thought came to dominate PNES treatment. Other psychoanalytic thinkers, such as Anna Freud and Melanie Klein, expanded on Freud's views and improved his theories by highlighting the significance of formative events in infancy and the power of the unconscious in influencing adult behavior.

While treating PNES, psychoanalytic treatment often entails assisting patients in identifying and exploring underlying psychological problems contributing to their seizures. There should be no judgment or criticism, just a safe space for them to speak about their feelings, relationships, and experiences from the past. The purpose is to educate patients on the causes of their symptoms and encourage the development of adaptive responses to stress and other precipitating factors.

Psychoanalytic theory, cognitive-behavioral therapy, and mindfulness-based approaches, to mention a few, are all supported by scientific data as effective treatments for PNES. Both the patient's goals and those of the treating physician should be considered while deciding on a course of treatment.

Therapies for PNES:

Psycho-education:

Psycho-education is an essential part of PNES therapy, but it is not a cure in and of itself. Those with PNES and their loved ones might benefit from psycho-education on the disorder's causes, symptoms, and treatment options. Individuals and their loved ones may better manage PNES and be more involved in their treatment if they have a deeper awareness of the disorder.

In addition to reducing the frequency and severity of seizures, psycho-education may help people notice the warning signals of an oncoming outbreak and build coping mechanisms to deal with stressful situations. Yet PNES can't be cured with only psycho-education.

Cognitive behavioral therapy (CBT), antidepressant medication, behavioral treatments, including relaxation methods or biofeedback, and collaborative care with a team of healthcare professionals are all potential components of therapy for PNES, in addition to psycho-education. Patients with PNES should collaborate closely with their healthcare team to create a personalized treatment plan considering their unique needs and goals.

Intrapersonal Therapy:

Due to insufficient research and clinical evidence about its efficacy in treating PNES, intrapersonal therapy is not routinely used as a therapeutic modality. Intrapersonal therapy, on the other hand, is a kind of psychotherapy that encourages patients to examine and gain insight into their minds and hearts to discover more adaptive coping strategies and overall better mental health.

Those with PNES who suffer from anxiety, despair, or trauma contributing to their seizures may benefit from intrapersonal treatment. Intrapersonal therapy can lessen the occurrence and severity of PNES by assisting people in recognizing and resolving the underlying causes of their distress.

Nonetheless, it should be stressed that psychotherapy is usually insufficient to cure PNES on its own. Cognitive behavioral therapy (CBT), antidepressant medication, behavioral treatments such as relaxation methods or biofeedback, and collaborative care involving a team of healthcare professionals are often used to treat PNES. If you or a loved one suffers from PNES symptoms, you must get help from a doctor with experience diagnosing and treating PNES. You may get assistance in creating a treatment plan that considers your overall health from their services.

Psychodynamic therapy:

Individuals with PNES may benefit from psychodynamic therapy, a kind of talk therapy, by delving into the roots of their symptoms and learning more about the unconscious processes at play. It is predicated on the idea that physical symptoms such as convulsions might manifest deeper underlying psychological issues originating in the individual's formative years.

Psychodynamic therapy has been proven successful in lowering seizure frequency and increasing psychological well-being in people with medically unexplained symptoms, including PNES. However, there is a lack of data on its application in treating PNES.

The hallmark of psychodynamic therapy is the weekly, one-on-one sessions with a trained therapist who provides a safe and supportive environment for clients to explore their thoughts, emotions, and experiences. The person may learn to cope with and resolve the underlying unconscious conflicts contributing to their symptoms via this procedure.

Psychodynamic therapy is not a stand-alone treatment for PNES; it is used with other methods, such as medication and cognitive behavioral therapy (CBT). Because of the complexity of PNES and the need for a tailored treatment plan, it's crucial to collaborate with a doctor with expertise in managing the illness.

Group therapy and Family intervention:

Individuals with PNES may benefit from group therapy and family interventions as part of their treatment because they may give social support, information, and practical coping techniques for living with the disease.

Individuals with PNES may benefit greatly from group therapy because it gives a safe space free from criticism where they can talk to others who understand what they're going through and get insight from their stories. As well as addressing any underlying psychological problems contributing to the seizures, group therapy sessions may concentrate on building coping methods, stress management techniques, and communication skills.

Family interventions may be helpful in PNES therapy because they educate loved ones about the disorder and teach them how to be there for the patient. Education on the disease, communication skills, training, and stress management and relaxation techniques are all examples of possible family therapies. Individuals with PNES may have greater feelings of support and agency when family members are actively engaged in their treatment.

The most successful treatment for people with PNES is multifaceted, including medication, individual psychotherapy, group therapy, and family interventions. Due to the complexity of PNES, it is essential to collaborate with a trained medical professional with expertise in treating the illness.

Therapists using Eye Movement Desensitization and Reprocessing (EMDR):

The original intent of Eye Movement Desensitization and Reprocessing (EMDR) was to treat traumatic stress disorders like PTSD. Among the mental health conditions that EMDR has been used to treat are ones characterized by somatic symptom difficulties, such as psychogenic non-epileptic seizures (PNES).

During EMDR, you'll move your eyes in specific patterns, which will help you process painful memories and lessen their emotional impact. In this method, the patient is asked to reflect on traumatic experiences while visually following the therapist's finger motions.

In paradoxical intervention, the therapist's use of humor, exaggeration, or other unexpected reactions disrupt the patient's maladaptive behaviors or thought patterns. When used effectively, paradoxical interventions may push individuals to alter their ways of thinking and doing.

Combining eye movement desensitization and reprocessing (EMDR) with paradoxical intervention effectively treats PNES and reduces seizure frequency and severity. Paradoxical intervention can help patients recognize the role of stress and anxiety in their symptoms and develop more adaptive coping strategies. But, EMDR may help patients deal with the trauma that's triggering their symptoms. Patients with PNES may benefit from a therapy strategy that combines EMDR and paradoxical intervention. Still, each person must get care personalized to their unique circumstances and symptoms.

Neuroimaging: What Is It?

In some instances, epilepsy may be traced back to alterations in brain anatomy. Hydrocephalus, scar tissue, and a tangle of blood vessels are all examples of such conditions (vascular malformation). Neuroimaging tests allow doctors to see inside the skull and determine if one of these diseases is present. Around half of the people with epilepsy have a definite explanation for their seizures; thus, these examinations are done to find or rule out other potential causes.

Standard neuroimaging for epilepsy often consists of computed tomography (CT) scans and magnetic resonance imaging (MRI). Both give an image of what the brain looks like. Compared to CT, MRI is preferred due to its greater diagnostic accuracy. MRI is the preferred imaging method.

Involvement of Neuroimaging in PNES Diagnosis and Treatment:

Stress and other negative emotions may trigger PNES, or psychogenic non-epileptic seizures, which are different from epileptic seizures since they are not caused by aberrant electrical activity in the brain. Neuroimaging modalities like

MRI, CT, and PET can aid in diagnosing and managing PNES.

To confirm a diagnosis of PNES, neuroimaging can help rule out alternative explanations for seizures. Imaging techniques such as magnetic resonance imaging (MRI) and computed tomography (CT) scans may detect structural abnormalities in the brain that may be the root cause of seizure activity. Differentiating PNES from epilepsy, which is also brought on by abnormal brain electrical activity, can be aided by this finding.

Neuroimaging also helps diagnose PNES by ruling out other potential causes of the patient's symptoms. For instance, evidence of a mood or anxiety issue may be seen on an MRI or PET scan, which might help direct therapy.

For therapeutic purposes, neuroimaging may help pinpoint brain regions that may play a role in PNES production or maintenance. Changes in brain activity linked to PNES may be detected using techniques like functional magnetic resonance imaging (fMRI). With this knowledge, we may create specific treatments that target the patient's unique psychological needs to alleviate the underlying causes of their seizures.

In sum, neuroimaging is seldom used alone to diagnose PNES; it may be a valuable supplement to other diagnostic approaches and give essential data for treatment planning.

What are the projections?

Proper therapy causes seizures to disappear in 60-70 percent of adults and much larger percentages of children and adolescents. Treatments for mental health issues are not a fast cure and need patience. Refusing the diagnosis and not moving on with therapy is a typical blunder.

Unfortunately, those who choose this course of action will keep taking antiepileptic medicines, notwithstanding their lack of efficacy.

Getting a proper diagnosis quickly is crucial. Patients have a higher chance of making a complete recovery if they don't have to live with a false diagnosis of epilepsy for as long as possible.

Stopping antiepileptic drugs should be done gradually (not suddenly) under a doctor's supervision if you have epilepsy.

Does my license let me drive?

After learning they have epilepsy, many people with PNES decide it's safer not to drive. Since specific laws do not govern patients with PNES, neurologists' opinions on whether they should move to vary widely. You and your psychiatrist or neurologist should make the call on whether or not you should be behind the wheel.

How about my disability?

This diagnosis should not affect any benefits you have been receiving or any time off from work you have been given due to your seizures. Whether epileptic or psychological, your attacks are pretty accurate and can potentially severely limit your daily life. Yet, if your neurologist no longer has authority over your care since your impairment is now due to PNES (rather than epilepsy), your psychiatrist or psychologist should take the reins.

The Benefits of therapy for PNES:

PNES treatments provide several advantages, including those listed below.

Better management of seizures: People with PNES who participate in therapy are more likely to learn to identify and regulate their seizure triggers, experience less stress, and increase their repertoire of effective coping mechanisms, all contributing to better seizure control.

The Quality of life enhancement: PNES may cause significant disruption in a person's everyday life, including absences from work or school, withdrawal from social activities, and other difficulties. Improvements in functionality and quality of life may result from therapy's assistance in symptom management.

Improved mental health: PNES patients often also deal with mental health issues, including despair, anxiety, and PTSD, so progress in these areas would be much appreciated (PTSD). Therapy can potentially enhance mental health and quality of life by addressing these root causes.

Self-understanding: People with PNES who participate in therapy report that they can better cope with their symptoms and make reasonable adjustments in their life due to the work they put into understanding their thoughts, feelings, and actions.

Improved relationship: Better communication and understanding between the person with PNES and their loved ones is essential. Strengthening interpersonal connections with loved ones is one of the many goals of therapy.

Therapy for PNES may be constructive for those who have this illness, leading to enhanced seizure control, quality of life, mental health, self-awareness, and interpersonal connections. You should consult a doctor specializing in PNES to figure out the best course of therapy for you.

Problems with traditional PNES therapy:

There are several problems with conventional treatments for PNES. There are many issues, but some of the most important include the following:

While psychoanalytic therapy has been the gold standard for treating PNES for many years, recent studies have shown mixed results. Some studies have demonstrated psychoanalytic treatment to be beneficial, while others have found no such effect for patients.

Access may be limited because of the high cost and lengthy duration of psychoanalytic treatment. In addition, access may be constrained by a need for more therapists with expertise in this method in certain regions.

People with PNES may face discrimination and misunderstanding from medical staff, loved ones, and the general public. Because of this, it may be hard for them to get the help they need.

Misdiagnosis as having epilepsy and subsequent treatment with antiepileptic drugs, which do not help patients with PNES, is a common mistake. Negative impacts and extra expenditures on medical treatment may result. Conventional therapy for PNES may not provide enough help in controlling the seizures themselves since they tend to concentrate on investigating the underlying psychological reasons that may be contributing to them. Patients may feel hopeless and frustrated as a result of this.

Considering these challenges, there is a rising interest in creating evidence-based, easily accessible, patient-centered therapy for PNES.

Advances in PNES therapy:

Many issues have been raised about the effectiveness of standard treatments for PNES. Notable matters include, but are not limited to:

Evidence-based therapy: Despite psychoanalysis' long reign as the gold standard in PNES treatment, recent studies have shown little to no improvement in patient outcomes. Some studies have demonstrated psychoanalytic treatment to be beneficial, while others have found no such advantage for patients to be gained by participating in the therapy.

Integrated care: Psychoanalytic treatment might be challenging because of its high price tag and lengthy recovery period. Further restricting availability is that there may be a shortage of specialized therapists in certain places who can use this method.

Misunderstanding and discrimination: People with PNES may face discrimination from medical staff, loved ones, and the general public. Because of this, it may be difficult for them to get the help they need.

Telemedicine: Misdiagnosis as having epilepsy and subsequent treatment with antiepileptic drugs, which are ineffective in managing PNES, is a common occurrence. Possible unintended consequences include increased medical expenditures.

Mind-bodies therapies: Conventional treatments for PNES may not give enough help in treating the seizures themselves, instead putting more emphasis on identifying and addressing the underlying psychological problems that may be contributing to them. Patients may feel hopeless and irritated as a result of this.

As a result of these issues, researchers have been more interested in creating evidence-based, readily available therapy for PNES to better patient outcomes.

Fields of study that contribute to PNES therapy:

Although neurologists and family doctors are often the first to be consulted to examine PNES, this is unsurprising given the symptoms that prompt the first visit. To make a correct diagnosis, a neurologist is essential. Patients are more likely to recover from their conditions if they are recognized and treated correctly early on. Frequent iatrogenic effects may be avoided by avoiding unnecessary repeat testing and procedures. An estimated 75% of PNES patients get AEDs before the correct diagnosis, which may lead to iatrogenic problems like those described above. The wrong diagnosis and treatment during interventions for extended episodes might be fatal. Evidence suggests that the longer a patient waits for a proper diagnosis, the worse their prognosis will be; however, this idea has lately been called into question.

Most medical doctors who diagnose PNES will send their patients to psychiatrists or psychologists for care since there are only so many effective therapies backed by solid scientific evidence. Even though a referral is the right course of action, no well-researched technique for facilitating this change in care delivery has been established. The low participation rates in treatment found in PNES may be attributed, in part, to the field's need for knowledge on the most efficient means of care transfer. Nevertheless, keeping the diagnosing neurologist involved is preferable so that AEDs may be tapered off safely, any new neurological symptoms, such as a shift in semiology, can be evaluated, and any co-morbid neurological disease can be treated.

It is recommended to begin working with mental health specialists throughout the diagnostic process. PNES assessment and management can benefit from the use of mental health services at three distinct points:

• During the diagnostic process, look for personality characteristics, environmental influences, and other medical conditions that may help explain the patient's psychopathology.

• When the diagnosis is given, which is an opportunity to get the patient interested in the treatment.

• During the administration of PNES-specific psychotherapeutic interventions.

Phases in PNES therapy:

PNES treatment usually consists of many stages; however, this might shift based on the specifics of each patient's condition and preferences. Some of the most crucial stages of PNES treatment are as follows:

Assessment: In the initial stage of PNES treatment, the patient's symptoms, medical history, and social functioning are evaluated. To determine the cause of the seizures, conducting a series of interviews, questionnaires, and diagnostic procedures may be necessary.

Education: When the evaluation is over, the therapist will usually teach the patient about PNES, including the disorder's causes, diagnostic methods, and treatment options. The patient's comprehension of their illness will increase, and their anxiety levels will decrease.

Treatment planning: The therapist will collaborate with the patient to create an individualized treatment plan based on the evaluation findings. This may need a multimodal approach, including talk therapy, medication, and behavioral modifications.

Symptoms management: Identifying triggers, learning relaxation methods, and building coping skills to cope with stress and anxiety are all examples of symptom management measures that may be taught to the patient as part of the next step of treatment.

Psychotherapy: Psychotherapy is helpful for many people with PNES because it allows them to address the psychiatric causes of their seizures. Techniques like CBT and ACT, as well as psychodynamic and other forms of treatment backed by scientific research, may be used.

Medication management: Some people with PNES may find relief from their symptoms with medicine. Nevertheless, antiepileptic drugs are ineffective in treating PNES and may exacerbate seizures. In this case, medication may be utilized to address comorbid illnesses like depression or anxiety.

Relapse prevention: The last stage of PNES treatment focuses on preventing a relapse, which may require continuing counseling, checking in with a healthcare practitioner often, and adjusting one's lifestyle to alleviate stress and anxiety.

Treatment for PNES is a team effort between the patient and their healthcare practitioner to alleviate symptoms and boost functioning.

Chapter 11

The effectiveness of drug treatment for PNES

Drug treatment for PNES

Psychogenic non-epileptic seizures (PNES) are not caused by electrical abnormalities in the brain but rather by emotional or psychological causes like stress or trauma. They can severely limit one's mobility and standard of living. Helping patients manage their symptoms and improve their health is impossible without adequate treatment.

One method of treating PNES is pharmaceuticals. Drug treatment for PNES is intended to improve quality of life by easing symptoms, decreasing the number and severity of seizures, and restoring normal brain function. In most cases, antidepressants, anxiolytics, and antiepileptics are used to treat PNES, all of which are side effects of the original medications.

Antidepressants, benzodiazepines, and anticonvulsants are some of the most frequently prescribed medications for PNES patients. Certain serotonin reuptake inhibitors (SSRIs) and tricyclic antidepressants (TCAs) have shown promise in reducing seizure frequency in several studies. Clonazepam and other benzodiazepines are often used to treat PNES because of their soothing effects on the brain and their ability to lessen the severity and duration of seizures. Because anticonvulsants like carbamazepine, valproate, and lamotrigine are so successful in treating epilepsy, they are sometimes used to treat PNES.

It's crucial to remember that not everyone will respond the same way to a given drug used to treat PNES and that results will vary from patient to patient. If the patient is to receive the most beneficial care possible, it must be tailored to their individual needs. In addition, psychotherapy and counseling should always be used with drug treatment for PNES.

Types of Drugs used in PNES treatment:

Psychogenic nonepileptic seizures can be treated with various medications (PNES). PNES medication is used to lessen the severity and number of attacks a patient experiences and to boost their overall quality of life. In most cases, antidepressants, anxiolytics, and antiepileptics are used to treat PNES, all of which are side effects of the original drugs.

Antidepressants:

In many cases, antidepressants like SSRIs and TCAs treat PNES. Despite their more common use in treating depression and anxiety, antidepressants help reduce the frequency and intensity of PNES episodes. Increasing serotonin levels in the brain are how SSRIs work, making them valuable in treating depression and anxiety. But TCAs are effective because they raise brain levels of norepinephrine and serotonin. These medications may not start working for a few weeks and may come with unpleasant side effects like nausea, dizziness, and dry mouth.

Benzodiazepines:

Commonly used benzodiazepines for PNES treatment include clonazepam. Because of their soothing properties, these drugs can lessen the frequency and intensity of seizures. Their effectiveness lies in amplifying the effects of GABA, a neurotransmitter linked to decreased anxiety and increased states of calm. Long-term use of benzodiazepines can result in drowsiness, dizziness, and confusion and can lead to addiction.

Anticonvulsants:

Medications like carbamazepine, valproate, and lamotrigine, known as anticonvulsants, are sometimes used to treat PNES in patients. These drugs are typically prescribed to those with epilepsy, but there is some evidence that they can also lessen the occurrence and severity of PNES. Specifically, anticonvulsants can prevent seizures by restoring regular brain electrical activity. Dizziness, nausea, and tiredness are possible adverse effects of these drugs.

Antipsychotics:

Seizures from PNES may be treated with antipsychotics such as risperidone or olanzapine if other psychotic symptoms like hallucinations or delusions accompany them. These drugs alleviate psychotic symptoms by preventing the brain from producing dopamine. Gaining weight, dizziness, and sleepiness are all possible adverse reactions to antipsychotic medication.

Medications' efficacy varies from person to person, and there is no magic bullet. If the patient is to get the best restorative care possible, it must be tailored to their individual needs. In addition, psychotherapy and counseling should always be used with pharmacological treatment for PNES.

Factors affecting effectiveness:

Drug therapy for psychogenic non-epileptic seizures (PNES) may be beneficial, although this depends on several circumstances. Among these are the patient's unique characteristics, the chosen medication (s) dosage, and any co-existing medical conditions.

- Factors unique to each patient, such as age, sex, and medical history, can impact the efficacy of drug treatment for PNES. Some patients may be less responsive to medications due to their history of substance abuse or addiction, while others may be more responsive to antidepressants due to depression or anxiety. In addition, higher doses or combination therapy may be necessary for patients with more severe or frequent PNES to achieve effective seizure control.
- How well a drug treatment program for PNES works can be significantly influenced by factors such as the medication chosen and the dosage administered. Some patients may respond better to a particular medication than others due to its unique mechanism of action or its lack of undesirable side effects. The severity of the PNES and the patient's response to treatment will determine the optimal dosage.
- Drug treatment for PNES may be less successful if co-existing conditions like depression, anxiety, or illness

are present. Patients with comorbid depression or anxiety may benefit from antidepressant therapy and other medications, and patients with comorbid epilepsy may require higher doses of anticonvulsants. Patients with co-occurring substance abuse or addiction may also need increased support and monitoring to improve the likelihood of taking their medications as prescribed and avoiding relapse.

- Cognitive-behavioral therapy (CBT), psychoeducation, and stress management techniques are effective psychological interventions that should always accompany drug treatment for PNES. These interventions have been shown to improve treatment outcomes for PNES by targeting the underlying psychological factors that contribute to the disorder.

- Individual patient characteristics, medication selection and dosage, comorbid conditions, and psychological interventions can all impact the efficacy of drug treatment for PNES. To ensure that each patient receives the most efficient and effective care possible, it is vital to tailor treatment plans to each individual's needs.

Limitations and side effects of drug treatment:

Pharmacological therapy for psychogenic non-epileptic seizures (PNES) is beneficial in reducing both the frequency and severity of these seizures, but it is not without risk. You and your doctor should discuss each treatment choice's risks and side effects.

The effects are minimal at best:

Although some research has shown that certain medications can help reduce the frequency and severity of PNES, no one drug or treatment will work for everyone. It's possible that some patients won't respond to medication or that they'll only get partial relief from their seizures.

Side effects:

Like any other medication, drugs used to treat PNES may cause unwanted side effects. Drowsiness, dizziness, nausea, weight gain, and changes in mood or behavior are all possible side effects. It's important to tell your doctor about any medications and supplements you're taking because some drugs can interact negatively with others.

Tolerance and dependence:

Benzodiazepines, one class of drugs used to treat PNES, can cause tolerance and dependence if taken regularly for a long time. When this happens, it can be challenging to stop taking the medication, and sudden cessation can cause withdrawal symptoms.

Comorbid conditions:

Many people with PNES also suffer from other conditions, such as depression, anxiety, or substance abuse, which can reduce the effectiveness of drug therapy. To get the most out of treatment, dealing with these root causes is crucial.

Psychological interventions:

Cognitive-behavioral therapy (CBT) and other stress management techniques should always be used with drug treatment. The problem is that these interventions aren't always readily accessible or covered by insurance, even though they're often quite effective.

Drug therapy may be useful for PNES, but it's important to be informed of the dangers and limits before starting. The most excellent likely results for people with PNES can only be achieved via a specialized treatment strategy incorporating pharmaceutical and psychosocial therapies.

Chapter 12

Life after Recovery from PNES

Emotions after recovery:

Several different feelings are possible after PNES recovery. Some of the feelings people have are listed here.

Relief: It's natural for people to feel relieved when they get a diagnosis and treatment plan for their epilepsy after battling for years with mysterious attacks.

Worry: Some people worry that their seizures may recur after recovering. They may be concerned about how the attacks affect their personal and professional lives.

Guilt or shame: Some people with epilepsy suffer guilt or shame because of the stigma and social isolation they may have faced due to their disease.

Fear of the Unknown: Healing from PNES may be a Protracted and Unpredictable Process. They may worry about what the future holds and whether or not they will be able to control their condition.

Gratitude: Feelings of gratitude arise when a person considers the help they got from others, such as medical professionals, loved ones, and friends, during their time of need.

Resilience: Those coping with PNES may gain strength and resilience as they face the many challenges of treatment and recovery.

Recognizing and accepting one's feelings is crucial for those overcoming PNES. Treatment from doctors, therapists, or support groups may also aid in emotional management and skill development.

Adjusting life without Seizures:

After overcoming PNES, learning to live a life free of seizures may be a significant life shift, but several coping mechanisms are available to aid people through this transition. Possible solutions are listed below.

- Putting one's needs first is an effective strategy for dealing with stress and enhancing health and happiness. Exercising, meditating, and other forms of relaxation are all examples.

- Gather a network of people who can provide emotional support by finding individuals who have been through something similar. While seeking help, finding a support group or therapist who can offer a confidential environment to talk about your emotions and get feedback might be helpful.
- If epileptic seizures were previously used to deal with stress or emotional anguish, the affected person might benefit from learning other methods. Some examples of such activities include discovering and exploring new ways to unwind, discovering and cultivating new areas of interest, and participating in new forms of creative expression.
- People undergoing rehabilitation may find it helpful to reestablish previous habits or build new ones that better suit their needs. Examples include rearranging one's job or school schedule, carving out time for self-care, or adopting a new set of healthy behaviors.
- Goal setting that is realistic and supportive of the rehabilitation process may be highly beneficial. This might help you feel like your life has meaning.
- Recovering from PNES may be emotionally taxing, so treating any mental or emotional health concerns that may crop up throughout the process is essential. Various treatments, such as talk therapy, medication, and surgical procedures, may fall under this category.

After PNES, it may take some time to adapt to a life without seizures, so be patient and supportive of yourself. Successfully adjusting to life without attacks is possible with the correct tools and approaches.

Building resilience:

Resilience training helps people recover from PNES by preparing them to deal with the inevitable setbacks they will face. Some methods to strengthen your ability to bounce back from adversity:

- To be aware is to accept one's thoughts and emotions as they are, without judgment, and focus on the current moment. It's been shown to help cope with stress, anxiety, and other mental and emotional obstacles.
- Concentrating on optimistic assumptions and ideals may help people become a more resilient and better deal with hardship.
- Mastering the art of problem-solving may equip you to face adversity head-on and emerge stronger on the other side.
- Develop a robust social network by spending time with loved ones or joining a group that shares your interests and concerns.
- Self-care should be prioritized as a means of stress management and resilience building.
- Learning how and when to reach out for assistance is crucial to being more resilient. One option is to visit a therapist, counselor, or mental health expert.

The development of resilience is not a one-and-done activity but rather a process that calls for consistent work and exercise. By implementing these practices into everyday life, people may strengthen their resilience and enhance their capacity to deal with difficulties during PNES recovery.

Moving Forward:

While moving ahead following PNES recovery, making some new, healthful resolutions might be helpful. You can help yourself and go on by doing these actions:

- Acknowledging and honoring one's development and successes may boost self-esteem and serve as a source of inspiration to keep working towards one's goals.
- It might be helpful to establish new objectives to get a renewed feeling of purpose and direction in life.
- Improve your physical and emotional well-being by incorporating healthy behaviors like frequent exercise, nutritious food, and restful sleep into your daily routine.
- Self-compassion is the practice of being nice to oneself and recognizing one's strengths, and it has been shown to increase both.
- Maintaining improvement and tackling persistent issues may be aided by consistently seeking assistance from healthcare experts, therapists, or support groups.
- Keeping oneself motivated and optimistic may be aided by adopting a positive mentality, such as reflecting on one's qualities and accomplishments.

Following PNES recovery, it may be helpful to take measures to enhance general health and well-being, establish fresh objectives, and adopt an optimistic outlook. Anyone may take steps towards a brighter future if they have access to the tools and resources they need.

Maintaining mental and physical health:

After beating PNES, keeping your body and mind in good shape for the rest of your life is crucial. Ways to keep your body and mind in good condition:

Frequent exercise: Exercising regularly has been shown to promote physical health and decrease stress and anxiety. At least 150 minutes of moderate-intensity exercise each week is suggested.

Healthy eating: Boost your health and vitality with a balanced diet of fruits, vegetables, whole grains, lean protein, and healthy fats.

Good sleep hygiene: Practicing good sleep hygiene, such as sticking to a regular bedtime schedule and making your bedroom dark and quiet, may improve your quality of sleep and your health as a whole.

Mindfulness practices: Meditation and other mindfulness techniques have been shown to positively affect physical and mental health by lowering stress levels and calming the mind.

Self-care: Putting yourself first by making time for hobbies or leisure is a great way to alleviate stress and boost your health and happiness.

Social support: Having a solid network of friends and family to lean on through tough times is an invaluable emotional and practical support source.

Counseling or therapy: Regular sessions help people feel supported and overcome difficult emotions.

Regular checkup: Checking in with a doctor regularly is a great way to keep track of your health and address any issues as soon as they arise.

After overcoming PNES, it is essential to continue participating in healthy behaviors and reach out for continuous help when you need it. Those with access to adequate tools and methods may sustain their health throughout time and advance in all aspects of their life.

Conclusion

In sum, PNES (Psychogenic Non-Epileptic Seizures) is a disorder that may have severe effects on everyday life and is often misinterpreted as epilepsy. The symptoms of PNES may be managed, and the quality of life of those who suffer from it can be enhanced with a correct diagnosis and appropriate therapy. Psychotherapy, cognitive behavioral therapy, stress management strategies, and medication for co-occurring mental illnesses are all often used to treat this condition. Individuals with PNES may learn to control their symptoms, improve their general well-being, and lessen the adverse effects of the disease on their everyday lives with the help of therapy and support.

www.ingramcontent.com/pod-product-compliance
Lightning Source LLC
Chambersburg PA
CBHW070553220526
45467CB00003B/1197